Looking at the STARS

Looking at the STARS

How incurable illness taught
one boy everything

by

Lewis Hine

Published by Lagom
An imprint of Bonnier Publishing
3.08, The Plaza,
535 Kings Road,
Chelsea Harbour,
London, SW10 0SZ

www.bonnierpublishing.com

Paperback ISBN 9781788702959
Hardback ISBN 9781911600770
eBook ISBN 9781911600800

A CIP catalogue of this book is available from the British Library.

Designed by Envy Design
Printed and bound in Great Britain by Clays Ltd, Elcograf S.p.A.

1 3 5 7 9 10 8 6 4 2

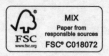

I would like to dedicate this book to all the doctors, nurses and healthcare professionals who have saved my life and supported me over the past 17 years

CONTENTS

'I love what Lewis has done with his life, it's so inspiring to hear. Giving him his Radio 1 Teen Hero award on stage at Wembley made me very proud, and hearing how loud the crowd screamed just showed what people thought of the amazing work he's doing. I saw first-hand the incredible things he is creating with Friend Finder when we worked on the prom together. Lewis is changing people's lives and he's a true teen hero.'

NICK GRIMSHAW

'To be comfortable in your skin was the biggest topic for me because I'm somebody who's always judged just by how I look. Lewis is showing the world it's OK to be different and that disabilities and personalities make the world colourful. Lewis said I'm his hero, well, he's mine. He is so young and going through so much just to stay alive and yet he gives his everything to help others and make a positive impact in the world. Keep fighting Lew.'

KID INK

'To me, in this day and age when we have so much bad news, it's so wonderful to see someone so young doing something so brave and so wonderful. It teaches us all a lesson. It's just really inspirational.'
ELTON JOHN

'Lewis continues to do incredible things in his life and constantly proves that one person can make all the difference in other people's lives, and for that I (and everyone else) am forever grateful.'
KSI

'Lewis is a true inspiration for us all to remember to never give up on our hopes and dreams – stay positive and keep fighting! I feel very honoured to support Lewis with this book that also raises awareness of epilepsy.'
JENNIE JACQUES
(QUEEN JUDITH IN *VIKINGS*)

Looking at the STARS

A BIT OF BACKGROUND
BEFORE YOU BEGIN

My NAME'S LEWIS, LEWIS HINE. I'm 17. I spend a lot of time sitting in my room playing Xbox games and watching films, and I can't leave the house without a responsible adult. Usually my mum.

I live just outside Portsmouth in a place called Leigh Park. It's the biggest council estate in the UK and, if you Google it, it comes up as one of the worst places to live in the whole of England.

Not long ago, my little sister Jessica and I were walking back from the Co-op when she nudged my arm.

'Hey Lewis, look at that,' she said.

I turned. This bunch of little kids was coming towards

us holding a plank of wood between them. They could only have been about eight years old, but the plank they were waving at us had nails sticking out of it.

'Hey!' they shouted at us. 'Hey, you!'

Then they started coming towards us.

'We're in trouble,' I said to Jess.

We were only about 15 metres from home but the thing is, I can't run. I've got epilepsy and every time I have a seizure my muscles get weaker. I have a lot of seizures – anything between 30 and 50 a week is normal, so there's no strength left in my legs. Half the time I'm in a wheelchair.

'Don't worry,' Jess told me, grabbing my hand.

She pulled me over the road and we made it across just before a white van drove past. That stopped the kids and gave us time to duck into our local corner shop. We went down the back aisle where all the cleaning stuff is and hovered about until we were sure the kids were gone. The bloke who runs the shop probably thought we were nicking something. There's a lot of shoplifting around here and there had been a nasty incident once when he'd suspected me. I'd gone in to buy some chocolate and when I picked the bar up, my hand clamped – that's an epilepsy thing too – so I had to balance it against my body. I was just trying to make sure that I didn't drop it, but the shop owner assumed

I was trying to put the bar in my pocket. There are a lot of misunderstandings when you're disabled.

And although I don't look disabled unless I'm in my wheelchair, I am. All in all I've had 13 life-saving brain surgeries so far, which means that my brain looks like Swiss cheese. All sorts of stuff has fallen through the holes, like my memory trigger and whatever it is that tells you when you need to wee. The epilepsy started when I was six, but I was diagnosed with a brain tumour and hydrocephalus, or water on the brain, when I was 17 months old. The surgeons managed to remove the tumour, but they couldn't cure the hydrocephalus. They've put a kind of tap in my skull for that; they call it a 'shunt'.

I go to the local college. I'm still doing maths and English because I failed my GSCEs, and I'm also doing a foundation learning course that includes a module called horticulture. That's gardening, basically. I hate gardening but the only other option was sports and, as you've probably guessed, sport isn't exactly my strong point. It's only a one-year course and I don't know if I'll pass anyway. It doesn't matter though, because I don't go to college for the education. I go because that's what normal kids do and so much of my life is not normal that I really enjoy the bits that are. Even if it means having to pretend to be massively into plants.

3

So college is OK and I actually like living in Leigh Park. Despite the odd wild kid, our neighbours are nice. People look out for each other. It's been home to me, Jess, my older sister Chloe, my mum Emma and our two dogs, George and Poppy, since I was a baby. Poppy's a Yorkshire Terrier and so is George officially, but we suspect he might actually be half wolf. He doesn't bark – he howls.

So in lots of ways I'm a pretty normal teenager and probably not someone you'd think would ever be asked to write a book. But I was. A woman called me saying she was a literary agent, and asked me to meet her. We had lunch in a cool burger bar in London and she talked about a hardback book with my face on the cover and my story inside.

If that sounds mad to you, it sounded completely insane to me. For a start, I can hardly write, because the muscles in my hands are too weak. But she'd seen the Facebook video about my life – I'd posted it on 17th March 2017 for my sixteenth birthday, and it went viral. She said I had a story to tell. And it turns out that you can talk a book into a digital tape recorder.

So I said yes. And I said yes for the same reason that I made the video: because I don't believe that disability is a bad thing. The bad thing is keeping silent about it. My life is a bit of a challenge. I'd be lying if I said

4

I never mind missing out on something because I've had yet another seizure, or that it doesn't ever bother me when someone asks me for the millionth time why I have a giant scar in the shape of a candy cane on the side of my head (it's where the surgeons cut through my skull to fit the shunt that drains the excess fluid out of my brain), but the truth is, I think I'm lucky.

When you're told you might die at any moment, every day feels special and it certainly means that we Hines don't sweat the small stuff. I did all the interviews for this book sitting in a camping chair in the sitting room, because the sofa Mum had ordered was six weeks late.

Mum finally called the company on 17th December.

'We have friends and family coming over for Christmas,' she explained. 'And I don't think Nan and Grandad would be very comfortable on fold-out chairs.' And she laughed.

The delivery man said, 'You're dealing with this very well. I'd be losing it by now if it was me.'

Mum just shrugged and replied, 'Well, compared to what we face every day, a missing sofa's not really top priority.'

She's right. Living with illness changes your perspective on life, and I think that's a good thing.

My physical and mental challenges also mean I understand how isolating disability can be, especially for children and young people who miss so much school that they can't make friends. That's what led to me launching my charity Friend Finder, and since that day in October 2015, Friend Finder has taken me on the most brilliant journey. I've met so many super-generous people who've supported the charity by donating money and time, and lots of incredibly strong people who are facing challenges much tougher than mine.

And I've done some really amazing things, like meet Prince William and Kate and go to the Royal Albert Hall to see the UK premiere of *Star Wars: The Last Jedi*. But best of all, I've been given the chance to tell my story and show the world that, while illness and disability might define the length of your life, they don't have to define *how* you live it. It's OK to be disabled. In fact, disabled people make the world more colourful. We can light up a room with our stories. I've written this book because I want everyone to know that by supporting each other we can all achieve what we want to achieve.

When we were trying to come up a title for the book, someone read me the quote 'We are all in the gutter but some of us are looking at the stars' (it's by the famous writer Oscar Wilde). I thought it was really cool. My take on it is that, no matter what stuff we have to deal with, we just need to think big and remember to look at the stars.

I hope you enjoy reading my story as much as I've enjoyed living it so far.

MR SPARROW
SAVES THE DAY

I WAS FIVE DAYS OLD when I made my first trip to Southampton General Hospital. It was a small thing, fixed in an instant with a pair of scissors. I had been born tongue-tied, which meant that the tip of my tongue was attached to that funny flap of skin underneath it so I wasn't feeding properly. The midwife spotted it, sent Mum and I along to the hospital for a quick snip and then we were home again. Sorted.

My second trip, 17 months later, was a bit less straightforward. I was only a toddler, so I don't actually remember any of this, of course, but Mum tells me that she'd been back and forth to the doctor with me for weeks because she knew there was something wrong.

My head was massive – so big I had to wear T-shirts made for five year olds – and I'd begun to regress; I'd stopped walking and started crawling again. The doctor said big heads ran in the family. It got to the stage where Mum was practically camped out in the surgery, but it didn't make any difference. They thought she was making a fuss.

Then one day we went on a trip to Longleat Safari Park for my big sister Chloe's birthday treat and apparently I just cried all day and kept banging my head with my fist. There's a photograph of me with Chloe; she's smiling her head off and I'm beside her with my dummy in my mouth, looking really miserable. You can see my eyes are bulging and my head is huge. Seriously big. I'm not going to lie; when I see it now, that picture shocks me.

Anyway, we got home and the next day Mum went round to Nan and Grandad's house in tears.

'There's something really wrong with Lewis, but no one will believe me,' she said.

She must have been in a real state, because Nan offered to take me to the doctor herself. Mum had just exchanged contracts on the house we live in now (we were moving from a two-up, two-down house around the corner, with no heating and a bathroom so tiny it had this extra-small bath you sat up in); so Nan told her to go round and measure up for curtains or something, as a way of taking her mind off things. Luckily for me, Nan saw a different doctor, who took one look at me and said, 'He has sunset eyes.'

Sounds pretty, eh? It isn't. It's when your pupils sink down, so more or less all you can see are the white bits. You look like a zombie, and it means the pressure in your head is so high that it's about to burst your eyeballs.

The doctor knew how serious it was straightaway. 'You need to take him to hospital right now,' she said. 'Have you got a car?'

Poor Nan and Grandad. They couldn't get hold of Mum, so they called my Uncle Mike and asked him to go round to the new house and fetch her in his car. I can just imagine it: there's Mum with her tape measure in her hand, chatting to the woman whose house she's buying when Uncle Mike turns up saying, 'Don't panic, but Lewis has been taken to hospital.' I bet panic's exactly what she did.

By the time Mum arrived at Portsmouth's Queen Alexandra Hospital they'd already taken me to the assessment unit to do a scan of my head. They did it with an ultrasound, which wasn't usually possible with a baby my age, but my head was so stretched that they could scan through the soft spot. When Mum was shown the scan she saw something that looked like a ball on the inside of my brain and her first thought was, 'My God, he's got a brain tumour.'

A doctor took her into a side room and told her to sit down. That's never a good sign.

'Have you heard of hydrocephalus?' he asked.

She hadn't.

'Well,' he explained, 'it's a build-up of fluid inside the skull, which can increase pressure and cause damage to the brain. Lewis has it, and if you hadn't got him here today, he could be dead in his bed one day very soon.'

Mum and I were bundled straight into an ambulance and transferred to the neurological unit at Southampton General. It must have been scary, but ask her about it now and she'll say she was actually quite relieved, because she'd thought I had a brain tumour and no one had mentioned that.

Her relief didn't last long. I had more scans as soon as I arrived, and these ones revealed that as well as all the water on my brain, I actually did have a tumour: a choroid plexus papilloma, to be precise, which looks a bit like a cauliflower. They're pretty rare, accounting for less than 1 per cent of all brain tumours and, to make matters worse, mine was in an unusual place. Most choroid plexus papillomas are found on the fourth ventricle, but mine was on the third, making it rare enough to get the medical staff excited. When I arrived in the high dependency unit, a whole bunch of students were brought in to look at me. It was my first taste of fame and I was too out of it to notice!

Mum was told that the best surgeon for an operation this risky was the amazing Mr Sparrow. Or Mr Crow, as Nan insisted on calling him. (It got so embarrassing that we had to ban her from being around at the same time as him.) I owe that man everything – he saved my life several times and when he removed the tumour, he even sewed my skull back together in a zig-zag so the hair would grow back better.

We had to wait a couple of days for him to be available. Parents aren't allowed to have a bed in the high dependency unit because of all the wires and machinery, so Mum just climbed into mine and refused to leave. She'd do exactly the same today, if it came to it.

She says the night before that operation was the worst of her life. I was pumped full of steroids and painkillers and kept being sick on her and she knew that there was quite a high chance that I wouldn't make it out of surgery. But I certainly wasn't going to survive without the operation. When the doctors came to take me down to the operating theatre, she tucked this white Andrex dog that had come free with some loo paper under my arm.

The operation took eight hours. It's hardly a spoiler to say I survived, but my heart stopped while I was in recovery. Mum, who'd been sitting outside in the corridor the whole time, saw the doors crash open and six people in gowns, masks and those weird Croc shoes run out pushing a bed. She couldn't see who was in it, but she caught a glimpse of the Andrex dog so she started running, too. When she was finally allowed in to see me she passed out. She was four months pregnant with my little sister Jessica at the time.

I feel sorry for my mum. I can't even imagine how hard it was for her to go through all that. And four weeks later we were back in hospital doing it all again. My fontanelle – the soft spot on the top of a baby's head – had never fused together after I was born and Mum had noticed that it was starting to bulge. (She learned later that it not fusing was a sign of a problem, but it had also helped to save my life because it meant that my head could swell; if it had been hard, my head would have burst under the pressure.) Another round of scans confirmed everyone's fears; the hydrocephalus was still there. Everyone had hoped that removing the tumour would cure that problem too, but I was unlucky I guess.

If you Google 'treatments for hydrocephalus' it tells you that the most common approach is the surgical insertion of a drainage system, called a shunt. That's what I've got. It means I have a valve behind my ear (it was made in a factory in Switzerland, where all the hi-tech watches are made), and a tube that goes from the valve down into my stomach to drain the fluid. It's a clever bit of technology and it keeps me alive, but like anything mechanical, it can go wrong. Blockages are the most common problem, but sometimes the tube slips out of the valve. This means that, rather than draining away, the fluid leaks everywhere. And the whole thing can get infected too – I have to be really careful about coughs, colds and mouth infections.

The first blockage occurred about three months after the shunt had been fitted. I recognise the symptoms now – I get a ridiculously bad headache, my eyes go a bit bulgy and then the pain gets so bad I literally can't move or speak – but back then it was just a case of Mum spotting that I was in trouble. Luckily, she was good at it, because if the shunt blocks, I have to have surgery within four hours or it's game over.

I get sent straight into a CT scanner when I go into hospital with a suspected shunt block. It's like a massive doughnut and I have to lie on a bed and have my head taped down to keep it still while the doctors do a scan of my head, neck and chest to make sure my shunt hasn't disconnected.

Any problem with the shunt involves brain surgery, but the X-rays reveal whether they have to go into my stomach, too, to sort out the tubing. It's like a hosepipe; sometimes it gets a kink in it. That's the worst part – worse than them cutting into my brain, because they have to go through all the layers of muscle, and afterwards I can't sit up. And laughing is really painful. I've had three stomach surgeries so far and each one has left me with a different scar.

I just needed brain surgery that first time. And the time or two after that, I think. To be honest, it's difficult to remember exactly when and why all the surgeries took place, even with all the photographs Mum took, because after a while they merge into one; but I'd certainly had five operations on my head by time I was five years old. The children's neurosurgery ward was as familiar as home.

On TV, hospitals are all drama and flashing lights, but the truth is that being in hospital is really boring. Mum was always inventing silly games to pass the time. My favourite was 'Guess the flavour of the chocolate', which involved taking a chocolate out of the box and guessing what was inside it without looking at the little menu thing. It's more fun than it sounds!

I had a lightsaber battle with Mr Sparrow one time, too. I was about two and a half and I was back on the ward recovering from an operation to fix my shunt. Mr Sparrow came round to see me with this massive team of students – he always had loads of students with him; they thought he was God. I was really into Star Wars at the time and I never went anywhere without at least a couple of lightsabers, so I held one up to him and said, 'D'you want a fight?'

To everyone's amazement, he nodded. 'Yes, I do,' he said, taking one of them off me.

We fought for about five minutes, me sitting up in bed in my pyjamas and him battling against me with his saber. The nurses ended up in hysterics and the students and other patients stared at us, amazed. Mr Sparrow was a leading brain surgeon, after all – a seriously important guy in a suit, and he didn't muck about. After that, whenever he saw me he'd say, 'Oh look, it's Lewis.'

I was lucky. My family were with me all the time, but I remember noticing that the boy in the bed next to me was always on his own. His head was so big that he couldn't even lift it off the bed to see what chocolate to pick from the box. I may only have been about three, but I could see that I had it pretty easy compared to most of the others on the ward. Yes, I was sick, but so were all the other kids I met, and at least I got to go home.

The two things I looked forward to each day on the ward were the daily trollies; one was filled with sweets and the other brought our food and was shaped liked a fire truck. Neither of them would have been possible without somebody raising money to pay for them. If you've ever spent any time in hospital you'll have noticed that all the nice things have been paid for with money raised by people doing brave, bold or plain silly things in return for donations.

That started me thinking. The idea that a three year old could wake up one day and decide to start raising money to help sick children sounds ridiculous, even to me, so most people assume that Mum was the driving force and I was just a cute figurehead. But it wasn't like that. In the world that I lived in, there were always new causes that needed money, and people were forever coming up with new ways to raise it. It was normal. I was just joining in.

One day I was at home with Mum and I said, 'Can we help the sick children too?'

She wasn't thrown by the idea. She just said, 'OK, what do you want to do?'

'Bowling,' I said.

I knew about bowling because I went with my godmother, Heather. She ran the local bowling centre and it turned out that the world champion trained there sometimes, so Mum asked Heather to pull a few strings. The next thing we knew, the bowling champion of the world had agreed to go head-to-head with me in a match in aid of the Association for Spina Bifida and Hydrocephalus (ASBAH, now known as Shine; spina bifida is linked to hydrocephalus). Mum helped me make some sponsorship forms and posters to put up in the bowling centre and the hospital (she and my sisters still do that stuff for me today – I couldn't do what I do without them), and about 100 people, including the local press, came to watch. I won, obviously, and I remember that everyone wore T-shirts with my name across the back, which was pretty cool.

Most of the events I did then were for ASBAH, but when I was five I organised a fun run to raise money for a special paediatric video unit that would help work out whether epileptic children could be helped by surgery. I had started school by then, so I persuaded 40 of my classmates to dress up in superhero costumes and run the Mini Great South Run. It wasn't difficult – what kid doesn't want to dress up as a superhero? (I was Superman, of course.) I gave them all sponsorship forms and they pestered their friends and family for money. Then the next day, 22 adults ran the full ten-mile course, also dressed as superheroes. I remember feeling a bit sorry for Buzz Lightyear because his costume was really heavy. The whole event raised over £2,000.

I did it again a couple of years later, only that time I

had to 'run' the 1.5km course in a wheelchair pushed by Mum, Chloe and Jessica because, by some weird coincidence, I had become an epileptic child myself.

My Top Tips for Life

★ My mum always says that she knew there was something wrong with me before I was diagnosed with a brain tumour at 17 months, even though the doctor said I was fine. She said it's called parental intuition – you just know if your child's not right. So if you're worried about something, keep pushing, and don't be afraid to speak to someone else if you're not getting anywhere. Don't be afraid to challenge the system. This applies to so many things in life, not just your health.

★ I started fundraising at three years old and people thought I was mad. They thought my mum was too. Don't let people's ignorance, or lack of understanding, make you change your goals. Explain what you're trying to do and just keep moving forward.

★ If someone you know is trying to achieve something, ask if they need help, or offer your support. I wouldn't have achieved anything without the support of my mum and sisters; they read and write for me, design posters, deal with the heavy legal stuff and help me get to places so that I can carry on doing what I do. This book may be about me, but there would be no book to write without my family. We're a team.

A Day in the Life:
22nd November 2017

4am: My head hurts – like, *really* hurts – and the rails on my bed are up, which makes it hard for me to get to the toilet without waking Mum, who's asleep on the floor. I don't think I've had a seizure as my muscles don't hurt that much, so I try to get to the toilet by myself.

4:30am: I manage to stand on Mum's foot as I'm getting out of bed and wake her up anyway. She says I did have a seizure about 11.30pm, and she was so tired that she'd just fallen asleep on the sleeping bag.

8am: Time to take my meds, shower and get ready for college.

9am: I meet my learning support assistant (LSA) in the canteen and say goodbye to Mum.

I'm pleased to be here. There are some great people in my class and we have a lot of fun. It was weird when I first started college, but now they all just think I'm funny – in a good way.

I have a time-out card that I can use in any lesson if I need a break or feel unwell. I try not to use it.

12 noon: I meet Callum and Jasmine from Friend Finder for lunch. Jasmine's just like Mum – she's always checking I've had something to eat or drink!

2pm: My head still hurts so the college secretary phones Mum to come and get me early. I'm meant to be here until 4pm.

6pm: I'm feeling better so I'm playing Charlie on Xbox Live. We're playing FIFA and I'm winning!

8pm: I have spaghetti for dinner with Mum and Jess, but I don't feel too good so I decide to go to bed and watch a film. Mum comes in with my meds.

11pm: I'm still awake but I'm feeling sleepy so I'm hoping for a quieter night.

2

SURGERY, SEIZURES AND HOLES IN THE BRAIN

ONE NIGHT I WOKE UP to find two paramedics standing at the end of my bed. They were wearing green uniforms and purple plastic gloves and, before I could realise what was happening, they'd put me in an ambulance and we were off to Portsmouth Hospital. I was six years old.

I don't remember anything else, but this is the story I've been told. Mum came up to my bedroom to check on me before she went to bed, as she did every night, and found me fitting in my sleep. She screamed, like mums do, and then called 999.

'I think my son's had a stroke,' she said. 'The whole left side of his face has gone all droopy.'

The operator was really calm. 'Go downstairs, open the front door and then go back up and stay with your son. The paramedics are on their way.'

They were at the house and in my bedroom five minutes later.

'It's not a stroke,' they said. 'He's had some kind of seizure.'

'He's got hydrocephalus,' Mum told them. 'He had a brain tumour and he's got a shunt in his head.'

That freaked the paramedics out. I was downstairs and in the ambulance before Mum had had time to ask our next-door neighbour to come and sit with Chloe and Jess. (Leigh Park may be a bit rough, but the community is solid. When there's real trouble, we help each other out.) We were in the hospital half an hour later.

It turned out that I'd had an epileptic seizure. Mum had been warned that epilepsy could be a side-effect of a brain tumour, but four years had passed since Mr Sparrow removed mine, so she thought I'd got away with that one. (In fact, the doctors said that the seizures had probably been going for ages before this big one, because I'd have these weird times when I just zoned out; but no one had thought much of it. That's the problem with having so many things wrong with you: there are loads of explanations for your symptoms.)

I don't think I was really aware of what was going on. I'd spent so much time in hospital anyway that I just accepted this as yet another admission, and the term 'epilepsy' didn't seem all that scary – you're diagnosed as an epileptic after a single seizure. It doesn't mean you'll have another one.

I have between five and seven a day, on average.

Seizures are like electrical short-circuits in the brain, and in my case, the worst ones, the tonic-clonic, happen mostly at night. They cause violent muscle contractions and I pass out – the type of thing most people imagine when they think about epilepsy. The convulsions are so powerful that they flip me right over. My pillow has special breathing holes in it so I don't suffocate, and there are guard rails on my bed. I only know when I've had one because I wake up with pulled muscles, or blood all over the sheets because I've bitten my lips again. I hate it when that happens. There's an alarm in the mattress that wakes Mum up when I'm convulsing. She doesn't sleep very well, I'm afraid.

A lot of people say that epilepsy is a hidden condition because your body doesn't show any obvious signs that you've got it. If I have a seizure in the street, which I do quite often, people think I'm just mucking about. That's the hardest thing, in a way.

The daytime seizures tend to be either random

twitches like a sharp, involuntary head turn, or just little absences when I lose track of where I am and what's going on. They happen so frequently that we've learned to be quite relaxed about them, and these days Mum only calls an ambulance if my lips go blue, or if the seizure's gone on for longer than five minutes.

There are drugs to control the seizures, of course, but it so happens that I have a very special sort of epilepsy that is drug resistant.

It took a couple of years of trials to work out that drugs didn't help. That was fun. The thing about these drugs is that they play with your brain and affect your mood. One particular combination turned me into a total psycho. I remember it really clearly: one minute I was normal Lewis and the next I started attacking anything and anyone.

One time I was at 24/7 Fitness, the gym where Mum helped out sometimes, and I went for this massive bodybuilder. I just walked up to him while he was doing some weights and slapped him on the head. He put the weights down, stood up to his full height and said, 'It's a good job I like you, Lewis.'

It certainly was. He was huge.

I kicked a nurse in the shins and once I even went for my nan. She'd come over to see us and Mum was trying to restrain me.

'You're overreacting, Emma,' Nan said. 'He's just a child. Let him go.'

'OK,' Mum said, 'but don't say I didn't warn you.'

Then she went into the kitchen to make a cup of tea. As soon as the door closed, I went nuts. I threw myself at Nan, punching and kicking. She managed to get hold of my arms and push me onto the sofa before I did any real harm, but it scared us both. I knew I shouldn't be doing it, but I had no control; it was like someone had taken over me.

'I'm so sorry, Nan,' I said, shocked at what I'd just tried to do.

'I know that wasn't you, Lewis,' she said.

We sat on the sofa together while we caught our breath, trying to make sense of it.

The next drug had no effect at all, so I was given another. Still nothing. Then the doctors added a third. This cocktail just made me feel really ill. I was drowsy and felt sick all the time, so Mum and I assumed there was a problem with my shunt. She took me off to hospital for some neurological tests – the ones where you have to do things like squeeze the doctor's fingers and hold your hand out flat. I failed all of them.

The EEG, which tracks and records brainwave patterns, revealed that I'd gone into something called 'non-convulsive status epilepticus', which basically means that a part of my brain was fitting non-stop. You could see this continuous spike of electrical activity on the EEG. It's really dangerous, so it was a no to those drugs too.

We've tried a couple of other epilepsy drugs since then and the ones I'm on now do help a bit (I know that because the doctors take me off them when I go into hospital for monitoring, and then I have massive seizures all day long), but fewer than five seizures a day seems to be as good as it gets.

Mum asked my consultant recently if my epilepsy was ever going to get better. She looked at me and said, 'Nothing is impossible. But no, I don't think it's going to go away.'

That was tough to hear, but I never give up hope – I even tried the ketogenic diet once because we'd heard that it could help. It didn't. Eating almost nothing but fat and protein just made my breath smell. I'm a possible candidate for surgery, but so far no one has found the precise area of my brain that's responsible for the seizures. But technology is improving all the time, and I'm due back in hospital for another round of 'monitoring'. There's a chance it will be what they call 'invasive'. I haven't had that before, but from what I've been told, invasive sounds about right: first they'll cut a trapdoor in my skull, and then they'll cover my brain with a mesh cap which I'll have to wear for a week (cool or what?). The hope is that someone will be able to pinpoint the miniscule bit of my right frontal lobe that's causing all the trouble. If that happens, the surgeons will be able to remove it and things might get a bit better.

I don't much like the idea of them taking out a chunk of my brain, if I'm honest, but it's a choice between having surgery that might, possibly, reduce the seizures, or carrying on as I am. Now I'm 17 I get to make the decision myself and I really don't know what to do. Obviously, I'd like to have fewer seizures, but every idea they come up with sounds even more lethal and scary than the one before. I'm keeping my fingers crossed that cannabis oil becomes readily available on the NHS soon. It's part of the cannabis plant, but it doesn't have the stuff that makes you high. My consultant says that trials carried out in other parts of the world suggest it could help control seizures, especially in young people with drug-resistant epilepsy like me. It's already been approved for use in America, so I may not have too long to wait.

When anyone hears about my medical history, they always focus on the brain tumour and the mechanical shunt in my head that keeps me alive, but in fact it's the epilepsy that's my biggest demon. That's what controls what I can and can't do in life.

31

These are some of the things I can't do:

I can't remember

My memory is tragic; so bad that I can barely remember my own name on a day-to-day basis. There are two reasons for this: surgery and seizures.

Brain surgery damaged my memory trigger, which means that although my long-term memory isn't too bad, I can't recall anything without help. Mum has made picture books of my life and filled the house with photographs, which all act as memory prompts. Without those, my life so far would be a total blank and I couldn't have told you any of the stories in this book. She had to sit in on all the interview sessions with boxes of photos and press cuttings.

My teachers use prompts too. I have a learning support assistant (LSA) with me in all my lessons and it's her (or occasionally his) job to give my memory a nudge with a key word. For example, if a teacher asks a question and I put my hand up, there's a good chance that I'll have forgotten what I was going to say by the time I'm picked. A good LSA will ask me to tell her my answer immediately, so when my memory fails she can give me a clue. Unfortunately, I'm not allowed any memory prompts in exams, which pretty much makes them a waste of time. How can anyone be expected to remember work they did a year ago when they can't even remember what they had for dinner the day before?

I was so fed up that I did a Facebook post about it after my GCSEs, and a woman messaged me back saying that she was a scribe who helped people like me take their exams. (A scribe sits with kids who have problems with their writing in lessons and exams. The kids talk and the scribe writes down what they say.) She said she'd often come across exactly what I described, and asked me if I'd be prepared to help her approach Ofqual, the exam regulation board. Obviously I said yes. So just before Christmas 2017, we got a letter back from Sally Collier, Ofqual's Chief Regulator, saying that the letter was 'receiving attention'. We're taking the fact that it wasn't a no as a real positive.

As it was, the only GCSE I passed was food tech because it's more coursework than exam.

The seizures wipe my short-term memory, which means that anything that happened in the hours before I have one is lost forever. It's made my school days an incredibly frustrating cycle of learning and forgetting – I'll sweat over a list of spellings or a maths formula then have a seizure, forget the lot and have to start all over again.

My memory – or rather my lack of it – is definitely my biggest challenge. We've developed all sorts of strategies to help. I used to have this Velcro ruler with pictures of all the things I needed to do that day stuck on it – everything from 'read your English book' to 'have a drink' – and I spent my childhood chanting rhymes and singing songs to try and make things stick. (We sang the times-table song so many times I think it's actually engraved on my brain.) These days I have alarms on my phone and I rely on other people a lot, too. At home, Mum, Chloe and Jessica make sure I'm up in time for appointments, that I've replied to an email or eaten my lunch; and I had the brilliant Mrs Ford at secondary school. She really had my back and was always going off to buy things I'd forgotten for lessons. She was especially useful in food tech because I was always forgetting to tell Mum what ingredients I needed. But the truth is that every seizure I have damages my brain a little bit more. And it's not going to get better. In fact, it's probably just going to get worse. Does that upset me? Yes, it does.

I can't be on my own

If I had to look after myself, I'd be dead within a day. All it'd take would be for me to have a little tiny seizure and walk into the road. Either that or forget to take my medication. I need 24-hour care and will do for the rest of my life.

At home that means there's a monitor in my bedroom, an alarm in my mattress and if I want to have a bath, I have to leave the door open and sing while Mum sits outside on the landing. It's a draughty experience and not very relaxing, so I don't bother very often.

At school – and now college – it means I have to have an LSA with me all the time, not just in lessons but walking to and from them, at break, lunch and when I go to the loo. It's partly because I can't remember where I have to be or how to get there (I managed to get lost in the school corridors on my last day at secondary school, even though I'd been there for five years!), and partly because I could have a seizure at any time.

Even the smallest seizure leaves me so out of it that I'm a danger to myself, but mine come with an additional hazard because I'm at very high risk of something called SUDEP. It stands for 'sudden unexpected death in epilepsy', and basically it means that when your heart stops beating because you're having a seizure (which it does), it doesn't start up again (which it should). So you die. Mum's known that I have this level of risk for years, but my doctors only told me when I turned 16. My first reaction was total panic, of course, but it doesn't scare me too much now.

I wear a wrist monitor all the time which sounds an alarm if my heart rate goes above or below a certain level. It's reassuring to know it's there.

I can't go on school trips or to other people's houses

If you're disabled you only get to go on the special disabled outings. At my school, that meant a day out fishing in East Meon every year. East Meon is a village about half an hour from where we live. I'm not really a fishing person, but it was quite fun (one year one of the kids managed to catch the science teacher), and there's a picture of me holding an enormous trout in one of Mum's albums. She says I got a prize for it.

You don't get invited to other people's houses either. Or I don't, anyway. My condition makes people nervous and I can't say I blame them; what with the seizures and the possibility that I might die, I am something of a liability.

Once, when I was about seven, my friend Stanley invited me to go swimming with him and his mum at the local lido. It was a hot day and Stanley's mum was sitting on the grass in the sun watching us play in the pool. It was a toddlers' one so the water only came up to our knees. We were mucking about, kicking water at each other, when apparently I just stopped and stood there in my armbands, completely rigid.

'Are you OK, Lewis?' Stanley's mum called, and rushed right over.

'My head hurts – really hurts,' I told her.

She grabbed her phone and called my mum.

'There's something wrong with Lewis,' she said. 'I'm bringing him home now.'

Then without stopping to get a towel, let alone change, she carried me to her car with Stanley jogging along beside us. Our house is only 20 minutes' drive from the lido, but I'd thrown up over the back seat three times by the time we got there.

Stanley's mum banged on our front door and Mum opened it to find her standing there in her leopard-print bikini with me in her arms, still wearing my trunks and covered in sick, while Stanley looked on in his armbands. We must have been quite a sight. Mum took one look at me and called the ambulance. I was having brain surgery for a blocked shunt two hours later.

After that, Stanley's mum was the only person outside the family who'd look after me. The way she saw it, the worst had already happened while I was in her care. How much worse could it get?

I can't tell when I need a wee

The bit of brain that tells me I need to pee doesn't work. I have an alarm so I don't wet myself.

I can't sleep in a normal bed

I sleep in a hospital bed, complete with rails to stop me falling out, a hoist so Mum can lift me and a motor that makes it go up and down. (Currently there's a giant hole in the wall behind the bed. That's where Mum managed to get the back stuck when she was moving it one time.) I spend a lot of time in this bed.

I can't drink alcohol

I'm 17 so I don't drink yet anyway, but I've been given the warning already. One beer could bring on a seizure. So could a Red Bull, for that matter.

I can't write or read well

As I said at the start, the seizures have weakened my muscles so much that I find it hard to hold a pen. I've missed so much school that I'm not that great at reading either. I like audio books, especially biographies of my favourite YouTubers like KSI.

And here are some of the things that Mum can't do because of what I can't do:

She can't work

She gets Carer's Allowance, and when I turned 16 she got a letter calling her for a review about going back to work. Mum was really excited. She said she would do anything at all but before she started, the council would have to provide 24-hour care for me. The interviewer crossed her off the list. (Now she says she works for me as CEO of Friend Finder, but I don't pay her. She's my mum!)

She can't sleep

My monitors and alarms mean that Mum can hear what's going on with me all the time, day and night. They keep me safe, but being constantly interrupted by electronic devices isn't very relaxing for her. (She does get her own back though; the monitor is two-way so she can speak to me when she's not in the room, and she likes to do ghost noises down it. They scare the living daylights out of me. One time, she spooked my support worker Matt, too. It was hilarious.)

She can't go on dates

Who wants to date someone who can't leave their disabled son? Recently I realised that I was so busy helping others make friends, I hadn't noticed that Mum gets lonely too. That does make me feel sad sometimes. Maybe I should put a post on my social media about her, like an advert, and find her a boyfriend. That would be really funny. She'd go mad!

It doesn't look great set out that like that and over the summer of 2015, I did get really low. I was 14 and I had this vision of me at 30, still living at home with Mum looking after me because I can't look after myself; we all know that that I'm not going to get better. I was due to have yet another operation, this time to change the programmable shunt (which hadn't agreed with me) to a fixed-pressure one. I remember wishing that there were two of me.

'I would like there to be two Lewis Hines,' I said to Mum one day, 'so I could be the one who wasn't ill. Then I'd be able to go out and have some freedom.'

I told the surgeon (a new one – Mr Sparrow had retired by then) that I didn't want any more operations.

'But it will make you feel better,' he said.

'You doctors are always promising that,' I replied. 'But nothing ever does.'

The truth is that at this point, I'd had enough of my life in general.

My Top Tips for Life

* Just because something has always been done a certain way, doesn't make it necessarily the right way. Don't be afraid to stand up for what you believe in.

* Every movement starts with one person. Be brave, be that person. It will be hard work and there will be days when you wonder whether it's all work and no reward, but if you stick at it, you'll make a difference.

SCHOOL

I'D HAD ENOUGH of school too. My memory issues mean that I have to work really hard to keep focused, so daily life is exhausting. I find it difficult to concentrate if there's a lot of noise around me, so the simplest things caused me problems. Like paying for lunch in the canteen – I couldn't work out how much my food was supposed to cost, so I wasn't sure if I had enough money to pay for it. It sounds daft now, but it didn't occur to me to ask for help and sometimes it was easier not to get lunch at all. (In the end Mum decided just to give me a £5 note every day but I used to forget to collect the change – I was the only person in the school to tip!) And as for lessons... well, I did my best, but when it takes all your energy to listen and you know you'll have forgotten everything five minutes later anyway, it's tempting to give up. But although it was a pain being tired all the time and struggling with lessons, it didn't really bother me. I wasn't going to school for the education after all. The reason I'd had enough was that I didn't have enough friends.

Primary school wasn't too bad. I went to a small Catholic school and when I started, I was pretty much doing the same as the other kids. I guess I was a bit behind, but not so much that my classmates really noticed. They noticed the scar on the side of my head, though (you can't miss it; it stretches from the nape of my neck to the top of my ear), especially when I went into school with new stitches. But when I explained that they were from another operation to replace or repair the shunt, the kids just nodded and accepted it. Small children are good at that.

Stanley was my best friend. He was a real character, quite full-on, but he was always there for me and he made me laugh. He came to visit me in hospital once. He turned up with this giant bag of cookies and chocolates and then, when Mum went out of the room, he climbed onto my bed and started playing with the controls. He put the back right up and we were sliding down it. We didn't know the room had a video monitor and that the doctor could see everything. Apparently he called the nurses and said, 'I think Lewis must be feeling better – he's hanging upside-down off the bed at the moment.'

Stanley came for a sleepover once, too, and I had a seizure and managed to wee on him. (I lose control of everything when I'm convulsing.) I only found out about that recently, when Mum and I were talking about him. It must have been gross, but Stanley never said anything to me – I think that's the mark of a proper friend.

He was pretty bright, so we went to different secondary schools, which made it difficult to keep in touch. We still message each other, even see each other sometimes, and when we do he still talks about that day in the swimming pool when his mum rushed me home in her arms.

Things started to get more difficult at school after the epilepsy kicked in. My seizures affect my balance, so I'd fall over a lot and bang my head, or just go all floppy and collapse. So when I was seven, the hospital gave me this helmet to wear to protect my head. I swear that helmet was the curse of primary school. It felt to me like it made the teachers really over-protective. They were so freaked out by the idea that I could smash my head and die that they made me wear it almost all the time – even when I was eating my dinner. Have you ever tried eating with a strap under your chin? It's tricky, to say the least. Mum had found me one of those padded rugby helmets, a slight improvement on the hospital's version, but even a cool rugby helmet only looks cool on the rugby field – in a classroom it just looks weird. Especially coupled with the headphones I had for when things got so noisy I couldn't concentrate. To be fair, the other kids never took the mick, but I hated that helmet and the headphones. I hated that they made me stand out and I hated that they made me look different.

I'd started to use a wheelchair by then, too. Not every day, but because a bad seizure can leave me too weak to walk, sometimes it was the only way to get me into school. And occasionally, I just needed it so that my body could chill out. I found school exhausting both physically and mentally and Mum soon realised that I had more chance of lasting the full day if I went in my wheelchair.

And that was important because I missed enough school as it was. My attendance fluctuated between 30 and 60 per cent, getting worse as I got older and the seizures and shunt problems became more frequent. I had a home tutor called Ruth who helped me a lot because she taught me visually – she did maths with Lego bricks rather than written numbers, stuff like that

– but I was struggling to keep up with the work my teachers were setting each day. And I was falling behind socially, too. I missed so much school that even though it was a friendly, small and supportive community and there were all sorts of measures in place to help me (I even had my very own quiet room to sleep in when I needed to), I began to feel more and more isolated.

Mum did everything she could to help, including throwing the most ridiculous parties for me. She'd save up for ages, invite the whole class and create these amazing themes around whatever I was into at the time. I was obsessed with the Power Rangers when I first started school so, for my fifth birthday, Mum got my uncles to dress up as the black and red Rangers; it was really exciting – you didn't see the Power Rangers walking around Portsmouth very often. I remember we had hot dogs, and Meridian News, the local ITV news channel, came. At the time, we were helping to raise money to keep an ASBAH charity advisor in our area, and everyone had donated the money they would have spent on a present for me to ASBAH instead.

I had a Star Wars party for my tenth birthday, complete with Darth Vader and a bunch of storm-troopers. I know now that Mum had somehow managed to hire the official George Lucas-approved UK Garrison impersonators, but we all thought the real characters had come. There were candyfloss and popcorn machines, and a chocolate fountain which one of the kids kept sticking her face into. There must have been 40 or 50 of us, including my classmates' brothers and sisters, and as the grand finale, we all walked through a tunnel of Star Wars characters before being presented with a lightsaber each by Darth Vader.

I know it sounds over the top, but when your mum signs at least one consent form each year that says there's a high chance that your son will die if he has this operation – and surgeons tell you he'll almost certainly die if he doesn't – then I suppose each birthday must feel like cause for a massive celebration. And I think she was trying to make me look cool in front of my classmates, too. I certainly needed her help.

We hired out a nightclub for my thirteenth birthday. I knew we didn't have much money and that Mum had to save up really hard for these parties, so I decided to write, with my sisters' help, to all these companies asking them to donate drinks and food. I just told it as it was. I said I'd had a load of brain surgeries, our family didn't have much money and I wanted to throw a big party for my birthday. The response was amazing. One company donated 1,500 bottles of soft drinks; others sent crisps and sweets and cake. I was really touched. We even got a DJ to come down from London after he saw a post asking for help with the music on my Facebook page.

So it was every 13 year old's dream party, right? Wrong. Yes, we had a food fight and shoved all the bottles of soft drink down the loos (what can I say? There weren't any bins and it seemed like a good idea at the time), but out of the 100 or so people there, about 90 were Chloe and Jessica's friends. I'd invited ten and only some of them had turned up. It's easy at primary school because your mum just invites the whole class and everyone comes, but at secondary school you have do the asking yourself and I only had a few friends to ask. It did upset me; it's not a great feeling to have so few friends that you need to borrow some from your sisters.

Part of the problem that year was that I'd missed even more school than usual. My shunt blocked twice, landing me in the operating theatre both times, and I also spent four or five weeks in Great Ormond Street Hospital having epilepsy investigations because my seizures had got really bad. (The investigations are horrible because, as I said earlier, the doctors have to take me off my medication. It's like going cold turkey; I have no control over my body at all and I shake so badly I can't even hold a cup of water.) I was away so long that my classmates assumed I'd moved to a new school and had forgotten all about me.

Secondary school was hell from the start. We were told that the local school, the one Chloe went to and where all my old primary-school classmates were going, wasn't the best option for someone with my disabilities, and that the best solution was for me to go to a comprehensive with a dedicated special needs unit. We knew that this school was at the bottom of the league tables, but they had a lift for my wheelchair, a physiotherapy room, a sleep room and lots of specialist staff who were used to dealing with kids with complex needs. Mum and I knew academia was never going to be my thing and, even though I wasn't in a wheelchair every day, this seemed like the safest choice. So we bought the uniform and off I went.

It was 45 minutes away by bus and I didn't know anyone.

If you're disabled, you don't catch the ordinary school bus. You get a special disabled one with an escort. My nan was the escort on my bus. Mum had arranged it – Nan was looking after kids on a different bus at the time, but Mum was so worried about how I would cope all by myself that she called the school transport department and asked if they could transfer Nan to my new school. It's not very cool, is it, having your nan on the bus, but to be honest, I was relieved. Stress tends to bring on my seizures and I don't think

I would have made it to school at all that first day if she hadn't been there.

I knew I was in trouble as soon as I arrived. The special needs kids were totally integrated into the main school and from what I could tell, I was the only one in my form. And everyone seemed to know each other already. I wasn't in my wheelchair – I'd been determined not to use it on my first day – but when I walked in, everyone turned to look at me. I just stood there wondering how on earth I was supposed to talk to these kids, let alone make friends with them. I knew they were looking at the scar on my head. I'd had my hair cut really short so that it wasn't as obvious, but there's no hiding it. I always tell people the truth when they ask what's wrong, and I was asked a lot of times that first day. Some of the kids were just curious. One, Charlie, came up to me and said, 'That's a really bad haircut, mate. I hope you got your money back,' which made me laugh. Charlie was OK. We did maths and English classes together and neither of us had much interest in the lessons, so we just messed about, chucking pencils at each other at the back of the class. He was my only friend in Year 7.

But some of the others used my scar as fuel to hurt me. 'You brain-damaged then?' was a question I heard a lot. There was no hiding the fact that I couldn't go anywhere without an LSA following me about, or that I had to eat my lunch in a special corner of the canteen, or that I'd come to school on a disabled bus. And by the end of the first week they also knew I used a wheelchair quite a lot of the time and that the escort on the bus was my nan. If anyone was looking for a reason to pick on me, they had plenty to choose from.

It was a rough school – I nicknamed it 'Fight Club' because pretty much every day somebody hit somebody else, and even the teachers were attacked sometimes. One had a mug of hot water thrown over her. It wasn't long before I got hurt. I was in a tech lesson and this boy, let's call him Elliot, glued my hands together.

'Come here, Lewis,' he said, grabbing me by the wrists.

I didn't see what he was holding and the next thing I knew, he was pushing my palms together. I could feel something hot and sticky. It was hot glue and it was burning my skin.

'How's that feel?' he laughed, pushing me towards his friend.

'What you need is a wash,' said the friend. We'll call him Kyle. He picked up a tub of paint and threw it at me, right in my face.

'Why the hell did you do that?' I shouted. I had paint in my eyes, my ears and up my nose and I couldn't separate my hands.

That got everyone's attention. The room went quiet – even Elliot and Kyle stopped laughing – and then my LSA rushed over and took me out of the class to get me cleaned up. The paint wiped off OK, but getting my hands apart? My God, I've never experienced pain worse than that. I'm surprised it didn't rip my skin to pieces.

Elliot was sent to the headmaster after that, because everyone in the class saw it happen and it's difficult to miss a multi-coloured boy who can't move his hands, but a lot of the things he and his friends did went unnoticed. I had an LSA with me all the time so they'd wait until she was distracted or helping someone else. Like the time I was punched in the face in a food tech lesson. This boy and I were at the back of the classroom clearing up, my LSA was sitting talking to the teacher – and the boy just went for me. I'd say it was totally random, but he'd disliked me from day one and had always used my disability as a reason to bully me. Some people seem to get a kick out of having a go at other people; I've no idea why. I can't remember if he said anything to me at the time, and I think I was probably too shocked to retaliate. I sometimes shouted at these kids but I never fought back – what would be the point? Fighting's never a good option for me; I'm not a ninja and I haven't got any reflexes. One punch and I'd get one straight back, twice as hard.

Mum told the head of year that I'd been hit, but nothing was done. None of the other 12 children in the room saw anything, and nor had the teacher or my LSA apparently. I suppose it could be true that they were all too busy washing up and chatting to notice a fight at the back of the room.

Soon after that, the same boy and one of his friends got hold of me. We were in class but the teacher was busy with another group. He pinned my arm to the table so I couldn't move while the other boy started cutting along the inside of my arm with a compass. He pushed so hard he drew blood. Mum found the marks when I got home and phoned the school immediately. They said they would ask around but when they called back, they said no one had seen anything – perhaps I'd got confused. Or I'd misremembered. It's true that my memory is unreliable, but I definitely had cuts on my arms and I know I didn't cut myself with a compass.

It happened time and time again. I'd come home with marks or bruises, Mum would call the school, they would promise to check and then we'd be told that no one else could verify my story. I began to wonder if I really was crazy. By the time I was in Year 8, a 'super-head' had been brought in – to turn the place around, we guessed. He was very focused on improving the school's reputation and we all know that reports of bullying are damaging.

Things came to a head for me in Year 10 when the boy who hit me in food tech started a Facebook group. He added a load of people from school and took a photograph from my sister Jessica's Facebook page (without her permission) to use as the group's cover photo. It was of me and her when we were really young on a Barney the Dinosaur ride.

It took me a day to realise what was going on. I'd been added to the group from the start, so I knew the picture was there. I wasn't all that bothered; the photo was a bit embarrassing – who wants to be reminded that they were once into purple dinosaurs? – but I was well used to people making fun of me. Then I started to scroll through the posts. One said that I should have been sent to Auschwitz, another that I should kill myself and save the NHS some money. I was so shocked that I just sat there looking at the screen in a daze. I knew they were saying it because I was disabled, but how did that mean I should *die*? I didn't get it. I just didn't get it.

Mum came in to my room and found me sitting staring at these messages on my TV. When she saw what I was reading she went crazy.

'This is disgusting, Lew,' she said finally, when she'd

calmed down. 'We need to report it. Don't you delete it, we need to screenshot it as evidence.'

So we let it play out for a few more hours. That was tough; the messages were really horrible. When we took the screenshots into school the next day, though, we were pretty sure that we'd be taken very seriously.

We weren't.

The school's response was that the messages had been sent outside school time and off the premises, so they couldn't do anything. So Mum went to the police. A couple of officers came round to interview me and the ringleader was charged with malicious communications. We agreed on something called 'community resolution', which meant the case didn't go to court and the boy wasn't given a criminal record. The police asked me if I wanted to choose what he did, but I said I didn't care. All I wanted was a letter of apology. When it came, it was obvious that his parents had written it. That really upset me, to be honest.

Charlie, my first friend at that school, stuck up for me. He refused to join the group, which was brave, considering he was one of the cool kids. Eden and Alfie were really supportive too. I'd met them in learning support in Year 8 and the three of us had clicked straightaway. We always made sure we had lunch together. Alfie was in a wheelchair, but he's done so much physiotherapy since then that he doesn't need it now. That's pretty inspiring.

But even with Charlie and Eden and Alfie around to talk to at school, I was finding it more and more painful to be there. I went because that's what normal kids do and I wanted to be a normal kid more than anything else, even if it was only for a few hours a day. But the bullying drummed it into me on a daily basis that I wasn't like everyone else. Every punch, every snide remark, reinforced the fact that I was different. They made me believe I was useless.

I began to withdraw, spending more and more time shut away in my bedroom, refusing to get dressed and inventing reasons not to go to school. At that point I believed that nothing would ever change for me.

My Top Tips for Life

★ Never try and guess what people think of you – it just makes you paranoid and will drive you insane. Do what you want to do in life and don't worry about what people think. Remember, you are amazing!

FRIEND FINDER
IS BORN

THE FIRST HALF of 2015 was rough. I felt really isolated; I had no one my own age to talk to and share my experiences with because I had so few friends. My older sister Chloe was bullied at school, too. That's her story to tell if she chooses, but one of the things she did to help her deal with it was to start campaigning. She'd applied for funding from GoThinkBig.co.uk, a youth development programme supported by O_2. GoThinkBig provides training and support for young people who want to lead social action projects in communities across the UK; they offer work experience and other opportunities as well. I'd been impressed by what Chloe had done, so at the start of that year I'd decided to apply, too. I went up to London and filled in the form telling them that I wanted to put on a party for children and teenagers who'd missed a lot of school and needed a way to make friends. I called the idea 'Friend Finder'. The grant was approved by O_2 in April 2015, a month after my fourteenth birthday, and I was sent a pre-payment debit card with £300 on it. Fantastic, right? You'd think so. But then the depression kicked in. Six months went by and the card just sat in my bedroom, doing nothing. Like me.

In June I had an operation on my feet – the most painful operation I've ever had.

I've had overlapping toes ever since I was a toddler – yet another side-effect of my neurological condition. I wore these big Forrest Gump boots at infant school, and then, luckily, when I went to junior school, the hospital gave me insoles to slot into my normal shoes. One was red and one was blue so I didn't get them muddled. They worked fine, but the condition got worse as I grew up. Before long I was treading on my toes as I walked, so it was decided that I should have an operation to straighten them.

Who knew that straightening your toes meant removing the knuckles and inserting metal poles instead? Certainly not me. You could actually see them – the metal poles, I mean. They stuck out of the ends of my toes and made me too scared to go anywhere in case they got knocked. They were like that for six weeks. The whole thing was horrific. Mum, Jess and Chloe called them my 'Wolverine feet', which looking back is quite funny, but I don't think I laughed a lot at the time.

The only thing I was really looking forward to was going to see Kid Ink. We'd got tickets to see him at the O$_2$ Guildhall in Southampton on 16th October. I am a massive Kid Ink fan and I'd saved up all my Christmas and birthday money that year so that I could buy some stuff from his Alumni Clothing line when we got there. I wanted a baseball cap (I collect baseball caps) and a chain with an A on it. As soon as I'd put them on, Mum took a photo and tweeted it. It said something like, '12 brain surgeries, a lot of pain. What makes Lewis happy? Kid Ink.'

Kid Ink saw it and retweeted it and the next thing I knew, there was a security guard standing next to me with his phone. We were sitting in the disabled area so we were pretty easy to find. We thought he was going to ask us to move, but then he showed me the tweet and said, 'Is this you? If so, Kid Ink wants to meet you after the show.' I couldn't believe it. We didn't expect him to even see the tweet, let alone do anything about it.

I was so excited that the gig passed in a blur. When

it was finally over, we were taken to a bar backstage. All the support rappers were there and Kid Ink himself was standing in front of this huge backdrop having his photo taken with people who'd probably paid a fortune to have a meet and greet.

'Wait here,' someone said. So we did.

One of the rappers was chatting Mum up.

'Damn, Mum, you're hot,' he said.

I mean, embarrassing or what? But Mum thought it was great, of course.

Then Kid Ink waved me over.

'Hey, Lewis,' he said. 'Take your hat off and I'll sign it for you.'

Then he put his arm around me like we were mates. I remember we were exactly the same height. He let us take loads of pictures – me with him, Mum with him; even Chloe and Jess had a turn.

Then his manager asked if we wanted any clothes.

'Wow, yes please!' I said.

The manager went away and came back with a pile of T-shirts.

'Here you go,' he said. 'On the house.'

Jess, Chloe and I were so shocked we just burst out laughing.

We were in there for ages – 20 minutes at least. What's that saying? 'Never meet your heroes'? Well, I disagree; Kid Ink was my hero and meeting him was one of the best things that's ever happened to me. The free T-shirts and photos were really cool of course but, more importantly, he went out of his way to talk to me and make me feel welcome. I was majorly depressed at that point, but the fact was, Kid Ink, a super-famous person, wanted to talk to me, Lewis Hine. He thought I was worth it, and that blew me away. As I left he said, 'You've got to keep fighting, Lewis.' I forget everything, as you know – and I've forgotten most of what he said that night – but those words really stuck in my head. By the time we got home, I'd decided that I'd take my consultant's advice and let them replace the programmable shunt with a fixed-pressure one, after all.

The problem with the programmable shunt was that because it was magnetic, it played havoc with the MRI scans. This meant I had to have X-rays before and after every scan to check the pressure levels hadn't been reset in the scanner. It caused a fair amount of chaos at school, too; I was in a science lesson once and we were doing an experiment with magnets, when I suddenly remembered that I wasn't supposed to be around magnets.

I put my hand up. 'I don't think I should be in this lesson,' I said. 'Magnets can interfere with my shunt.'

The poor teacher went as white as a sheet.

'You need to get out, Lewis, straightaway,' he said.

Then he ran over to where I was sitting, picked me up and literally carried me out of the classroom before I even had a chance to move. Everyone except him thought it was hilarious.

Meeting Kid Ink gave me the push I needed to put my Friend Finder plan into action, as well. I decided to use the O_2 money to pay for a Halloween party for kids in my area whose illnesses made it hard for them to make friends. Kids who looked different, behaved differently, or who had just spent so long in hospital or at home in bed that their classmates had forgotten all about them. Kids like me, in other words.

I put posters in schools and community centres, hired out the local leisure centre, bought a load of Halloween decorations and ordered a huge stack of takeaway pizzas, garlic bread and potato wedges. I had no idea how many people were going to come because the adverts and Facebook posts said to just turn up, but I didn't want anyone going hungry. (If you're wondering how a 14 year old with no memory and writing like a four year old did all that, then the answer is, of course, with help. I had the ideas and dictated the emails. Mum, my sisters and their friends did the organising. They were like an army of personal assistants.)

There's always a horrible moment just before a party when you worry that no one will come. I remember standing in the Havant Leisure Centre sports hall with this huge fake scar across my forehead, next to Mum in her devil horns and Jessica, Chloe and a bunch of Chloe's friends all dressed up as ghosts. The place looked pretty good – there were inflatable ghouls, paper pumpkins and a ton of food, but I was sure I'd made a mistake. Perhaps there weren't any other kids like me.

But there were. One by one, 20 kids, ranging in age from four to 16, arrived in fancy dress. They bobbed for apples, bounced the inflatable ghouls around the hall and ate every potato wedge on the table. It was fun. But the weird thing was, they didn't talk to each other. The younger ones just stayed with their parents or carers and the older ones hung around with the people they already knew.

I had expected people to be shy – that's normal. It can be tough, introducing yourself to a stranger. But I'd given everyone a pencil case containing a piece of paper and a pen so that they could exchange phone numbers and email addresses with the people they met... and no one was using them.

It didn't take me long to figure out why. All these kids had a disability of some kind, and had missed a lot of school. I knew all about that, and what it does to you – you end up with poor social skills, zero confidence and you probably can't read and write very well, either.

The result of this little mix? Isolation. No wonder no one was swapping contact details. It suddenly dawned on me that these kids were struggling with exactly the same issues as me, and that our shared problems gave me a unique perspective: I understood exactly how they felt. Watching everyone at that party made me realise that they were so like me that I really could do something to help them.

A couple of years earlier, I'd gone to a trade show called Event Tech Live with Mum. She'd volunteered to help a friend out, but I was going through a rough patch; she didn't want to let her friend down, though, so she decided to take me with her. (She dressed me up in a jacket and tie and pretended that I was on work experience. I'm not sure we convinced anyone – it was obvious that I was feeling pretty bad.) It was really dull standing about on her stand all the time, and at one point I wandered over to the booth opposite that was demonstrating this cool gadget called a Poken. It's a hand-shaped USB stick that uses near-field communication to allow people to swap information simply by touching two together. When you plug it into your computer, it brings up a photograph of everyone you connected with and if you click on the photo, you get that person's contact details.

I was given a free sample to take home, but as I

didn't know anyone else with one, I just stuck it in my drawer and forgot all about it... until those unused pens and paper at the Halloween Friend Finder party got me thinking. That was it! I could make it much easier for people to exchange contact details! I wrote to the company who made Pokens, but they didn't reply. I couldn't think of a better product for Friend Finder so I wrote again, this time sending it straight to the CEO. Looking back, I'm quite surprised that I had the guts to do that, but I think I was so determined to make Friend Finder work that I didn't stop to wonder whether a 15 year old should be writing to the head of a company asking for favours. I explained that I was launching a project to help isolated children make friends, and that I thought Pokens would be a really valuable tool. My cheek paid off: a few weeks later 250 of them arrived at my door.

I knew they would be a real game-changer. Giving members of the Friend Finder family Pokens not only meant they wouldn't have to admit they had problems reading and writing, and all that embarrassing stuff; these cool little gadgets would also give them a reason to go and speak to each other in the first place. There's nothing like a new piece of tech to get people talking!

I couldn't wait to try them out. It was December, so I thought we'd have a Friend Finder Christmas party.

I got chatting to a man called John at a car boot sale; when I told him about Friend Finder, he offered to let us have the party in the community club he ran. It had a bar, a juke box and a snooker table so it was the perfect place for a teen gathering. Mum bought a Christmas tree, but John and his staff gave us everything else for free, including the pizza and chips. Charity projects depend almost entirely on goodwill, and there were a lot of people like John in my community. For example, one of our neighbours messaged me on Facebook to say he had a signed Pompey football shirt (Pompey is what everyone calls Portsmouth Football Club) and would I like to offer it as a raffle prize to raise some money? Local businesses supported us too – the Car Finance Company made a donation and all the staff volunteered to help out at our events. I couldn't have got Friend Finder off the ground without that kind of help. People can be amazingly generous.

About 30 teenagers turned up to the Christmas party and we gave each of them a Poken. They went down really well. Mum's got this video of the evening and you can see everyone touching their Pokens together, exchanging details. Afterwards, one of the parents said that she'd found them really helpful too because, rather than waiting for her son to tell her who he'd met at a party (which he never did), she could see their names on the Poken and that meant she could help make sure they kept in touch.

Seeing Friend Finder working made me feel so much better, physically and mentally. School still wasn't the best, but at least the bullying had eased off. When the boy who'd started the Facebook group received his community resolution, it had shocked everyone. Even at my school, the kids were quite frightened of the police.

But before I could do any more I had to go back into hospital to have my programmable shunt changed. To be honest, I don't like to think about what the surgeons actually do when they operate, but Mum says that for this one, they had to open up my head and my stomach and join the catheter in my stomach to the connection point in my head. I was pretty sore afterwards and although I was only in hospital for three days, I was dizzy for about a week. You tend to feel a bit concussed when you've had people fiddling about in your brain.

Once I was back on my feet, I started to put my plan into action. The first thing I had to do was find some money. I'd spent the initial £300 grant from O_2 on the Halloween party, and although Mum had paid for decorations at the Christmas party, she certainly couldn't afford to fund anything else. I knew O_2 also supported longer-term projects to help young people grow and scale up their ideas, so I went back to the team at GoThinkBig and applied for the year-long grant of £2,500. My proposal was to put on one Friend Finder event every month for 12 months.

The great thing about GoThinkBig is that they don't just give you the money. If they like the sound of your proposal, they invite you to attend a series of workshops in London. Each one focuses on a different aspect of setting up and running a project, from budgeting to marketing. We almost missed the first one because we didn't realise how far the venue was from the tube station. We started walking, but I was in so much pain I had to sit down. Mum called the team at O_2 and said, 'I don't know quite where we are but we can't get to you.' Five minutes later this man appeared with a wheelchair. I've no idea where he found it, but it made my day.

The sessions themselves were pretty daunting because everyone was older than me and none of them had a disability. I had to take Mum along to help me remember what I needed to say – and I don't think they'd ever let a mum in the room before. The worst bit was when we all had to stand up and give a five-minute talk about our idea. I'd never spoken in public before and here I was having to stand up in front of 80 strangers. It was terrifying. I didn't have anything prepared, so I just told my story and explained that

I wanted to launch Friend Finder to help other kids like me. This woman at the back of the room was in tears by the time I'd finished. I was worried I'd said something to upset her, but Mum said she was just moved by my story.

The training process may have been hard, but it was also incredibly useful and by the time the money came through on 2nd June 2016, I had some idea, at least, of how to make my Friend Finder dream a reality.

Top of the 'to do' list was to find a venue for the monthly parties. I'd had the Halloween party at Havant Leisure Centre so I decided to try there first. They were really supportive, so I booked one of the sports halls from 4pm to 6pm on the first Thursday of every month for the next year. Having an official Friend Finder slot for our social events made it all feel very real.

Marketing was next on the list. The publicity campaign began with designing a website. I say 'design', but what I mean is that me and a couple of family friends called Max and Jack used one of those website-building tools and just stuck pictures and text all over a luminous yellow background. It was tragic. The text wasn't even inside the boxes on the mobile version. The site may have been rubbish, but at least friendfinderofficial.com was live. (I'm pleased to say that Mum has redone it since, and by the time you read this there will hopefully be a proper one designed by someone who really knows what they're doing.)

There's a story behind the web address too. When we first typed 'Friend Finder' into Google, a load of porn sites popped up, which really isn't what you want for a site aimed at disabled children. Mum wrote to one of them asking whether they would put up a black 'adult content' front cover, and she even offered to buy one of the other sites, but none of them got back to us. So we decided to add the word 'official' to our name; it's not ideal but at least it seems to have solved the problem.

I also made friends with *The News*, Portsmouth's local paper. They had covered some of my fundraising events in the past and were really supportive from the start. They would write short pieces about what Friend Finder was doing each week and print the website and email addresses. That publicity was incredibly important. Friend Finder only succeeded because the local community got behind me and, at least in the early days, the local community only found out about what I was doing because of *The News*. I owe them a lot.

The first of the regular monthly Friend Finder events took place on Thursday 7th July 2016. It had a sports theme and I hired a bouncy castle. That was a real winner – even the older kids were jumping around on it, including me. You'll often find a bouncy castle at children's parties and school fetes, so most kids have grown out of them by the time they reach their teens; but the people who came to this Friend Finder event had missed a lot of parties while they were growing up. A bouncy castle was still something to get excited about.

Putting on an event for disabled children isn't like hosting a normal kids' party because there are so many safeguarding issues. Mum has had a Disclosure and Barring Service (DBS) check, which proves she doesn't have a criminal record, and Matt from the leisure centre volunteered to be our first-aider, but it was a steep learning curve. I managed to get hit with a basketball at that party – someone threw it down the room and it bashed me square on the side of the head. I don't think my ears are any more delicate than anyone else's, but it hit me so hard that it burst my eardrum. I couldn't hear properly for weeks. It's quite funny really; I've never been allowed to do sports and then I start organising sports events for Friend Finder. We were so focused on keeping everyone else safe that we let our own guard down.

I'm happy to say that no one other than me has been hurt at a Friend Finder event, but I do seem to be a bit accident-prone. We went to the Hemel Hempstead Snow Centre once; taking 22 disabled kids skiing takes some planning, I can tell you, but with the help of

Snowbility, we did it. There were autistic kids, a boy with one leg, someone with a catheter and another with a terminal brain tumour – and things didn't go so well for me. It took half an hour to get me into the sit-ski and, although I set off facing forwards like a normal person, I somehow managed to spin round 180 degrees and finish my descent backwards. I've never seen so many people run away from me. It was terrifying.

To be fair, not everything we do with Friend Finder is physically dangerous. Some of the events are just socials – a chance for kids to hang out together in a place where everyone feels safe and comfortable enough to be themselves. It sounds like such a simple thing, but when you've spent a lot of your childhood in hospital, or your entire school career feeling different, it's the normal things, the stuff that everyone else takes for granted, that you miss out on.

There are quite a lot of older teenagers in the Friend Finder family and I wanted to put something on for them that would give them a taste of what it's like to go out with their mates for the night. I hired a bar with a snooker table and a darts board and we all just hung out. There wasn't any alcohol, of course, but for most of the people there – me included – the experience of ordering even a lemonade from a real bar was enough of a treat.

Friend Finder has grown massively since those early

days, but it changed me as a person right from the start. I'd reached a point where I couldn't go on without having a friend – after all, it's one of the most basic things in life. Everyone needs someone to talk to, to have a laugh with and create memories with. By launching this project, I made myself a whole new family of friends. To be honest, I find setting up the events quite stressful because organisation is not one of my strong points, but seeing people arrive with hardly anyone to talk to and then leave two hours later with multiple new friends and contacts makes it all worthwhile. Seeing so many people looking happy and just being themselves around other people makes me feel really pleased with what Friend Finder has achieved.

There are currently over a million kids in the UK suffering from a long-term disability or illness that keeps them away from school. Lots of healthy kids might think it sounds great to skip school, but take it from me, the reality over long periods of time is that you get lonely. School might be a bit boring sometimes, but it's also full of kids – it's the place where young people learn how to communicate and play with others. It's where we learn how to make friends. I set Friend Finder up to help people who were missing out, like me. And by doing that, I helped myself out of my depression. I feel incredibly lucky.

My Top Tips for Life

★ If you're being bullied like me and my sister Chloe were, tell an adult. It doesn't matter who – it could be a teacher, a parent, an aunt, uncle or a youth worker in a club. Just make sure you tell someone. You may think you're saving them from a problem by not telling them, but you're not.

★ If you're a parent worried about your child because they're acting differently, talk to them so they have a chance to tell you what's up.

★ If you know your friend is being bullied, don't just stand there and watch. Tell an adult. OK, it's scary, but you must be brave and let people know what's going on. They will help you.

★ If you can't find an adult to tell then call Childline on 0800 1111. They're trained to help you deal with what you're going through, and they're amazing.

★ More disabled people get bullied than any other demographic. There are no excuses for bullying, of course, but one of the reasons it happens is that people don't understand disability. We need to share our stories and be proud of who we are. The more we do that, the less ammunition they will have to use against us.

★ Remember, the bully is probably going through something challenging, too. Often, later in life, they really regret their actions and what they did plays on their minds. Even if you are an adult who feels this way, send the person you bullied a message saying sorry, because it's never too late to apologise. And it may help you to finally put the bad feelings behind you.

✱ I used Friend Finder to help me when I was being bullied. I found out about O$_2$ GoThinkBig and contacted them to get involved. If you're being bullied, or are feeling down, look out for groups you can join in your local community; it will help you feel better. There are lots of big companies who support community projects so, if you have an idea, don't be afraid to contact them and ask for their help. No matter what age you are, this is a great way to forget the bad and focus on the good. Trust me, I've done it and it works.

HELLO, WEMBLEY!

MY PHONE RANG one day at the end of August 2016. I didn't recognise the number.

'Hello,' I said, half-expecting it to be one of those spam calls where someone tells you you've been in an accident that wasn't your fault.

'Is that Lewis Hine?' the voice asked. 'This is Radio 1.'

I thought it must be some sort of joke, but I said, 'Yeah, this is Lewis.'

'I'm calling to tell you that you've made it into the final 30 for the 2016 Teen Awards,' the voice said. 'You were nominated by your mum and we need to make sure you're happy to go ahead. It's a huge deal if you win. You have to go on stage at Wembley Arena in front of 10,000 people, live on Radio 1, for a start. And there will be media attention too.'

Well, I was shocked. Mum's always been my biggest fan, but she hadn't told me she'd put me forward. I'm not sure I really took in much of what they said to me after that, but I did know that this kind of opportunity wasn't going to come my way again.

'Yeah,' I said, still unable to believe what I was hearing. 'That's fine.'

Mum had come into the room by then.

'Who was that, Lew?' she asked, when I hung up.

'Radio 1,' I replied. 'They wanted to know if I was happy about being nominated for a Teen Hero Award because I've made it to the final 30.'

'And are you?' she asked quite seriously, as if it had nothing to do with her.

'Yes,' I said. 'It's cool. Thanks.'

'Oh Lew,' she said, and came over to hug me.

I was glad Mum hadn't asked me beforehand, because there's no way I would have let her send off the form. It seems a bit big-headed, doesn't it? You know, like, 'I've done something so heroic that I (rather than one of the thousands of young people doing brave and good things in the UK) deserve an award.' But now that she had, I was really excited. We all were.

We were told that the winner would be announced on 19th September, but the day came and went and nothing happened. The next day we were in Asda choosing cereal when Mum's phone rang. She answered, then went all quiet, and passed it to me.

'It's for you,' she said. She had this funny expression on her face like she was trying not to smile.

'Hello,' I said.

It was a man I didn't recognise. He said, 'Hi Lewis, this is Nick Grimshaw. From Radio 1.' As if he needed to add that. I listen to his show all the time. 'Congratulations, you've won. You're a Radio 1 Teen Hero.'

I was so surprised, I literally couldn't say anything. I just dropped the box of Shreddies I'd been holding and passed the phone back to Mum.

'He's thrilled,' she told Nick, and started to laugh.

I'm not going to lie, we did a little dance right there in the cereals aisle in Asda. We didn't give a monkey's what anyone thought of us!

Three weeks later, Mum and I were staying in a posh hotel in London courtesy of the BBC. They took us to see the *Charlie and the Chocolate Factory* musical in the West End, then on a tour of the Radio 1 studios. The other winners and shortlisted kids were there too. Niamh was the other Teen Hero. She runs an online support group for young people with chronic illnesses because she's had multiple health problems since she was born, and was bullied so badly at school that she got depressed and started self-harming. Alex and Carys, who are both young carers, were the shortlisted heroes and then there were Joe and Toby and Lauren and Lucy. Joe and Toby got the One Million Hours Award for the fundraising they'd done in memory of their friend Arran, who'd died of a brain tumour, and Lauren and Lucy won the Make it Digital prize. They'd been part of a team who had come up with an idea for a lightweight medical kit called the Medical Military Shuttle, and Lauren and Lucy had then gone on to inspire other girls to follow their lead. They were a really amazing bunch and I felt proud to be there with them.

After the tour we had lunch with all the DJs who'd been on the panel – Nick Grimshaw, Scott Mills, Clara Amfo, Chris Stark and Greg James. That was exciting enough, but then we were told that we were going to spend the afternoon at Kensington Palace. With Prince William and Kate.

The journey there was really funny. Nick Grimshaw, Clara Amfo and Greg James were travelling in this luxury minibus with us and when we stopped at the traffic lights on Oxford Street, all these people started banging on the windows. I knew they weren't interested in me, but I felt really famous anyway. And then the next thing I knew I was walking into the palace. I don't think I'd believe it had happened if it weren't for the photo, but there it is: Nick Grimshaw, Clara Amfo, Greg James and Lewis Hine of Leigh Park, Portsmouth, about to walk into Kensington Palace.

Someone – a security guard or maybe even a butler, they must have one of those – showed us through the front door and my first thought was, 'Oh my God, their house is massive.'

Mum was taken off for tea somewhere and the rest of us were shown into this huge room. I remember noticing that there were loads of family photographs all over the place. Nick and I headed straight for the back where the biscuits were. Then Greg came in.

'Guys, attention please,' he said, and in walked the Duke and Duchess of Cambridge. Kate was wearing this long white dress with red flowers all over it.

'This isn't a dream, it's really happening,' Alex whispered in my ear.

That's exactly how I felt too.

'I don't know how you all find the time to do the volunteering,' Kate said to us all. 'It's such a great thing. Keep it up.'

'Yes, massive congratulations,' said William. 'Seriously impressive.'

Nick and I were still munching on the biscuits and

I thought that would be it, but then Clara said, 'This afternoon has been a perfect way to let our Teen Heroes know just how valued they are,' and started introducing William and Kate to each of us. I stuffed my half-eaten biscuit in my pocket.

'This is Lewis,' Clara said, and first Kate and then William shook my hand.

William said, 'You have people looking up to you and saying that you are a shining light for your age group.'

That made me feel a bit weird. Stress has a nasty habit of bringing on my seizures, and meeting the heir to the throne, however nice he is, is about as stressful as it gets. So, of course, I had one. Not a big one, just one of the small, twitchy face sorts, but it was noticeable on the video Radio 1 made for the Teen Awards website. The whole left side of my face gets pulled up so it looks like I'm making a face at him. I also zone out completely while I'm having a seizure, which he must have found a bit strange. William and Kate were both far too polite to say anything.

Then Greg stepped into the middle of the room.

'We have some badges that we'd like you to distribute,' he said, handing a silver tray piled with little black boxes to William.

William and Kate went round the room again, handing

each of us a box with a bright yellow Radio 1 Teen Awards badge inside it. I'm happy to say that I did manage to speak this time. 'I'm really happy to receive this,' I said finally. 'It's come as a bit of a shock.'

William just smiled.

Once we'd all got our badges, William looked at us all. 'Thank you, Radio 1, for doing the Teen Awards,' he said. 'It's fantastic to highlight all you champions. You're a huge inspiration. I know you are the most modest people I have ever met, but you should be proud of all the hard work and effort you're putting in. You're leading the way. Well done.'

We had the royal seal of approval!

Afterwards, Greg said, 'It doesn't really get any better than that, does it?'

I would have agreed, except that I got to stand next to Kate in the photo.

But in fact, all that was nothing compared to the Teen Awards ceremony itself. Meeting Kid Ink the year before had shaken up my ideas, and helped me to stop feeling sorry for myself and do something positive with my life; winning a Teen Hero Award gave me a springboard to make what I'd started bigger and better than I'd ever imagined. And it was great fun, too.

It's impossible to describe what it feels like to walk out on the stage at London's SSE Arena, Wembley in front of 10,000 screaming teenagers. But on Sunday 23rd October 2016, that's exactly what I did.

I heard Nick Grimshaw say, 'We welcome on to the stage the one and only Lewis!' and then someone gave me a shove. As I walked through the Radio 1 arch into all these light beams and heard the crowd screaming, I raised my hands in their air like I was some kind of superstar. I have no idea why I did that – everyone else had been really low-key and modest. I think I was just enjoying myself. Nick put his arm around me and handed me this big green disc with a giant 1 cut into it. 'This is Lewis, everybody,' he said. 'Congratulations. How does it feel to finally get your Teen Award in front of 10,000 people?'

'It's crazy,' I told him. 'It's something I never thought would happen. It's just been completely surreal.'

There was more screaming.

'Has it been loud enough today, d'you think?' Nick asked.

'Yeah, I'm probably going to go out deaf,' I said. 'But it's all cool.'

'All cool,' laughed Nick. Then he turned back to me. 'I just wanted to say, on stage, that what you're doing is so incredible. It's such a cool idea, so congratulations from me and everyone at Radio 1 and everyone here at Wembley.'

I thought that was it, but he went on. 'You're a bit of a gamer, aren't you? So we've got a message from someone that I know you're a big fan of. Check this out.'

The screen behind us came to life, and there was the YouTuber KSI.

'Hey guys,' he said, 'it's your boy, KSI.'

Even I was screaming now.

'Radio 1 has sent me a video of your amazing, awesome story,' KSI continued, 'and it just completely blew me away so I thought, you know what, we definitely need to get together, get the controllers and go head-to-head. I'm not going to go easy on you, so you might like to get some practice in.'

I literally couldn't believe what I was hearing.

'All right, so that's going to happen,' said Nick. 'It's going to be KSI versus you, Lewis.'

'That's a bit of a battle,' I replied, 'and I don't know who's going to win, but I think it'll be KSI – I'm not as good as him.'

Nick laughed. 'Well, what we've done – and we don't want to take sides, but we want you to win – is we've got you some amazing gaming things that we're going to give you so you can practise.' He paused. 'And since you're here and you're such a gaming fan, do you want to present our Best Game winner?'

I nodded, thinking that things couldn't get any

weirder. He told me to press this button, then the whole of Wembley did a countdown and Nick said, 'And the winner is Pokémon Go!'

A massive Pikachu walked onto the stage. The problem with Pikachus is that they don't have proper hands, so I just had to pretend to give it the award.

There was a photo session too. All the Teen Hero winners had to stand on this red carpet while loads of photographers shouted, 'Over here please! Teen Heroes, look to your left! This way please!'

By the time it was all over, my head was spinning. Mum had said she'd take us out for some food and I was really ready to eat, but when we got to the stage door, a security guard stood in our way.

'Don't go out there,' he warned us.

'Why not?' I asked. 'We're going to TGI Fridays. I'm starving.'

He opened the door just wide enough for me to see. I'm not joking – there were about 200 people standing out there, and all I could hear was, 'Lewis! Lewis! We want Lewis!'

It was insane. I laughed, but the truth is, I was petrified.

Obviously, we couldn't stay inside Wembley all night, and after about 20 minutes it was clear that the crowds weren't going anywhere either. The security guard let us out.

'Run for the hills,' he called, as the crowd spotted me.

There were shouts of, 'There he is – Lewis! Over here! Lewis!'

'I think they're really taken with you, Lew,' Mum said, laughing as groups of people rushed over to ask for selfies.

The security guard was keen to move us on. 'If you hang about for photos you'll block the pavement,' he said in this really serious voice.

But now I was outside, I was quite enjoying it. Everyone was really friendly. One guy in a pink T-shirt came up to me and said, 'Can I get a picture with you? You're a real inspiration. Well done, mate.' How nice is that?

It didn't stop even when we finally made it to TGI Fridays. It seemed like everyone there had been at the Teen Awards and they all wanted a picture with the award winners. I didn't even manage to have a sip of my drink. It was a crazy night.

The next day I was back at home in the real world (there's nothing like sisters and seizures to keep you grounded) but, although it might sound a bit big-headed, when I looked at the award on the shelf in my room, it did make me feel proud. And it gave me a massive spur to keep going and to work harder. I knew that winning this award wasn't an end – it was a reward for a job done, yes, but it was also a new beginning. It was an amazing platform that I could use to make Friend Finder bigger and better, and to make sure everyone has a friend.

Oh, and in case you're wondering what happened when I went head to head with KSI, like most things in my life, it didn't turn out quite how I'd expected. I did get the gaming stuff Nick had promised, but the match itself was cancelled. I wasn't that surprised – the whole thing had felt a bit mad anyway. Then on 2nd January 2017, I was just lying in bed when this huge guy in a black hoodie walks into my bedroom. I was so shocked I didn't register who it was for a minute. Then it clicked. It was KSI.

'No, don't do that to me!' I exclaimed, getting up.

'What's up, bro?' he said, cool as anything.

'Ah dude, you scared the living daylights out me,' I said, laughing. 'Normally I'd expect my mum to come through the door.'

'No, just me, bro.'

Yeah right – like KSI walks in my bedroom every day.

'How's it going?' he said. He started rummaging about in his bag. 'I come with gifts. I've brought quite a few. I wasn't sure whether you were an Xbox or PlayStation guy, so I got you both. And some chocolates.'

Games and chocolate – it was like he knew me already.

Then he said. 'Your house is quite a long way from Kent.' It turns out that he'd come all the way in a taxi. I couldn't believe it – it must be 100 miles.

Mum ordered some pizza and then we had our match. He beat me at FIFA but I got him on UFC, so I call that a draw.

My Top Tips for Life

★ Don't do something hoping you'll be paid back in return. The universe has a magical way of balancing things out. Acts of kindness are often returned to you in the strangest ways when you least expect them. When you help someone, whether it's by volunteering, caring or creating, do it just for the sake of helping them and making a difference to their life. The reward is that it will make you feel really warm and gooey inside, and believe me, that's a great feeling. Anything else is a bonus.

★ Take a chance. I had no idea what reaction I'd get when I walked out onto the stage at Wembley Arena. I was taking a big risk, waving my arms in the air and enjoying myself. But I did it. And it felt great.

★ Oh, and if KSI ever turns up at your house to play Xbox, make sure you play UFC, because he's really good at FIFA!

A Day in the Life:
30th December 2017

4am: I have a bad headache. Mum's asleep on the floor of my room so I guess I've had a seizure. It's horrible not being in control of your body, but it's worse not knowing what's happened. I go back to sleep.

11am: I only just woke up. I must have been tired. Mum's just come in and raised the bed and given me my medication. She's given me some tea and toast as well.

11:15am: My head still hurts so I'm staying in bed now, watching *The Fast and The Furious*.

12 noon: Mum's gone to the shop and Chloe's looking after me.

1pm: Mum's back. She's made me some lunch, just a chicken and bacon sandwich and a protein yoghurt, so that's going to be my food for the day. She's going to help me eat because all my left side is weak today.

2:30pm: Mum says I need some fresh air, so I take my wheelchair to go to the shops. I really want a new Xbox controller but I know

Mum can't afford it, so I'm paying for it with the money I've saved.

3:30pm: I've just got home and I'm going to try out my new controller. This is what I spend a lot of my time doing, just sitting here playing on my Xbox.

4pm: I pause the game because I've got to have a Skype meeting with Charlotte, who's helping me write this book.

4:45pm: I couldn't do as much work with Charlotte as usual today because I'm so tired, but I tried my best. I'm knackered now.

6pm: I'm in bed with a headache. Mum tried to give me dinner but I'm not hungry.

8pm: I'm watching *The Hitman's Bodyguard* in bed. My mum is sitting on the end of my bed watching it with me. My sister Jessica is upstairs with tonsillitis, so Mum's running between us.

12:15am: I guess I've been asleep, as my sister Chloe has just come in from work and the dog's barking woke me up. Mum's voice comes through the monitor, scaring me, but I guess she just heard me move and wanted to check I was OK. I'm going back to sleep now.

THINKING BIG

I WAS READY to do something big. Really big.

Sitting on my bed a few weeks after the Teen Hero Award, I posted a message on Facebook asking everyone in the Friend Finder family to name one thing they would really love to do. I don't know what I was expecting, but it certainly wasn't 'Go to a prom'. But that's what came up, again and again.

Of course, once I stopped to think about it, it was obvious; the prom is a major topic of conversation from the moment you start secondary school. It's a rite of passage for every 16 year old. Or every 16 year old who's well enough, confident enough and able-bodied enough to be able to go to school. Unsurprisingly, lots of the people involved with Friend Finder were going to miss out on their school prom.

So that was it. Decision made: I was going to organise a Friend Finder prom for all those teenagers who had missed – or knew they would miss – their own. It would be like the other Friend Finder events, just bigger and with dresses. Or so I thought.

I went back to Facebook and asked for volunteers to help me 'plan a big project' that would take place at Portsmouth Guildhall on 2nd June 2017. If it all sounds a bit cloak-and-dagger, that's because I didn't want too many people knowing what I had in mind, especially so early in the process. I got a pretty good response; 20 adults and teenagers said they'd get involved, but when it came to it, only four turned up for the first meeting. That was a bit disheartening.

And while I wasn't getting far with helpers, Mum was using my new Teen Hero celebrity to try to persuade TV production companies that it would be a good idea to make a documentary about this amazing prom I was organising. Talk about blagging it. But it turns out that she's a good blagger and on Christmas Eve 2016, CBBC agreed.

I spent almost the whole of January 2017 in hospital having tests and treatments so, by the start of February, we still had nothing more than an over-ambitious idea and a TV crew anxious to start filming. We had two major problems: first, our £15,000 fundraising target was still just that – a distant target – and second, the 'army of volunteers' we'd mentioned to CBBC was actually a bunch of disabled teenagers with no experience of organising anything.

I did another shout-out for volunteers, without mentioning the documentary. I knew I'd get more people if I did, but I didn't want anyone to be part of this just because they saw it as a chance to get their face on the telly. I only wanted people who were genuinely interested in helping Friend Finder achieve its goals. Five adults and eight of the Friend Finder kids – Callum, Eddie, George, Hannah, Jasmine, Eden, Billy and me – turned up for the next meeting. We became the planning committee.

I'd like to say that we were strategic, and allocated certain jobs to certain people depending on their skills, but we really weren't. It was a more a case of jumping in with both feet and keeping everything crossed. We asked the local supermarket if we could go and offer to pack people's bags at the checkout one Saturday. We'd seen other people raising money doing that. The supermarket manager said yes, but when we got there I'm sorry to say that most of the customers were really vile. We'd tell them that we were raising money for the Friend Finder Prom and ask if we could help them pack their bags, but most of them gave us the death stare and said no. They probably took one look at my shaking hands and assumed I'd break their eggs (which I probably would have done, to be fair). Some fundraising leaves you feeling you've really achieved something, but after a day of that, we just felt like we'd wasted our time.

We tried car-washing too, and a neighbour called Julia offered to do a day's face-painting. She did the painting and I sat next to her in my wheelchair with my little bucket and a bunch of Friend Finder posters. We were there from 9am until 4pm, but by the end we'd only raised £70. At that rate, it was going to take us 215 days to raise our target; we only had about 100 left until prom day.

I knew we needed help. I contacted the leader of Portsmouth City Council and asked if we could meet – after all, I reasoned, Friend Finder was providing a service for disabled children in the area, and the council would surely want to support that? I went with my sister Jess and was just really honest; I said that we had this great plan for a prom, but that we were literally on the edge with no money, despite our fundraising efforts. The councillor made a one-off donation of £1,000 there and then. That was a huge help – not simply because it was a large injection of much-needed cash, but also because it made our GoFundMe page look better; people are reluctant to donate to a cause that hasn't secured any funding.

Portsmouth City Council also gave us a space to use as Prom HQ (it was the lower ground floor of the multi-storey carpark, but what it lacked in glamour it made up for in convenience – it was opposite the Guildhall), offered to pay for the red carpet and gave us the square outside the Guildhall free of charge. It's not easy admitting that you need help, but I'm so glad I did – their support changed everything.

I was determined to have a red carpet and to give everyone their moment of fame as they arrived at the Guildhall. My original plan had been to have it leading up the steps outside while spotlights arced across the sky in true film premiere style, but once we'd measured it all out, we discovered a hitch: an outdoor red carpet's meant to be attached via some holes in the steps, but they'd been accidentally filled in and we would have to pay to have them drilled out again. So the carpet went inside.

That wasn't the only compromise. I knew that how you arrive at prom is almost as big a deal as what you wear, and I had this idea of hiring a fleet of supercars (I'm a massive supercar fan), which would be parked outside the Guildhall so that everyone coming would have a chance to sit in one and have their photograph taken. The council agreed, but in the end there was simply too much for our small, inexperienced team to do; the reality was that if the prom was going to happen at all, we needed to concentrate on the basics.

Like music. We really wanted a live band and had this wish list of A-listers – Ed Sheeran, Adele, The Vamps, Matt Terry – written on the wall at the office. Of course, we had no idea how to go about finding a band, let alone a super-famous one, so I decided to ask someone who did. I still had Nick Grimshaw's number in my phone from the Teen Awards and, after a lot of fretting and some encouragement from Mum, I wrote him the following message on WhatsApp:

> 'Hey Nick, do you remember me? It's Lewis from the Teen Awards. I need some advice on the planning of the massive prom I'm organising. Thanks from Lewis.'

I sat on the sofa with Mum while she willed me to send it.

'Are you really going to do it? Go on, you press it,' she said.

'Here we go.' I hit send and looked up at my mum. 'Done.'

We stared at the screen together. 'Oh my God, it's got two ticks, it's actually arrived,' she said.

'Crazy! What am I doing?'

'I can't believe you've just texted Nick Grimshaw asking him for help,' said Mum, giggling. 'OK. If he doesn't reply, don't worry. People must ask him for help all the time, so let's not get too excited.'

I sat there for a serious moment, thinking. Then: 'Hey, yeah!' I said, throwing my arms up in the air. We lay back on the sofa and laughed.

I was convinced Nick wouldn't even remember who I was. He must meet hundreds of new people every month.

But he did remember. A few hours later I was in the kitchen with Jess when a text came in. It said, 'Hey Lewis, great to hear from you. That sounds fun. Why don't you come to Radio 1 one day and meet us and chat through some ideas?'

I couldn't believe it. A few days later I was sitting in a big swivelly chair at the Radio 1 studio telling Nick Grimshaw all about our plans. He was incredibly enthusiastic – although he did point out that major pop stars' diaries are 'insane... actually they work like dogs, they literally work every single day!' So the chances of getting Ed Sheeran or The Vamps to play at a prom in Portsmouth were quite slim.

When he saw that I was disappointed, he said, 'The night needs to focus on the people going there and the reason why they're going. They're going to experience the prom they missed out on – you don't want people asking for tickets so they can see a star perform.'

It was probably the best advice anyone gave me.

Nick offered to help us find an up-and-coming band, and suggested that we ask people coming into Radio 1 in the weeks leading up to the prom to record a message of support that we could broadcast on the night. The roll-call of celebrities walking through those doors is impressive, and before we knew what had happened, we'd had shout-outs from the likes of Olly Murs, Emeli Sandé, Rita Ora, Clean Bandit, Niall Horan, Jess Glynne, KSI, Louisa Johnson, Two Door Cinema Club and even The Vamps. And we also had the very brilliant indie singer Jerry Williams lined up to play. She's from Portsmouth, too, which was good.

We also needed clothes. I didn't want money to be a barrier at my prom, so everything was going to be free. That meant we needed enough dresses and suits and pairs of shoes for everyone – with spares so there was a choice of styles and sizes. Jasmine put a post on Facebook asking for anyone with an old prom dress to get in touch. It was shared over 300 times and suddenly Prom HQ began to disappear under a mountain of silk, sequins and tulle. It was exciting – until we discovered that every dress needed cleaning and that we didn't have any clothes rails to hang them on. I remember we had one meeting where we couldn't see the floor for dresses, so everyone decided to put one on – even the film crew. (I'd like to make it clear that this didn't include me; the girls tried, but I wasn't having any of it.)

And we needed guests: 150 of them, plus a carer each. (The room could hold 350 but we capped it at 300 to make room for all the wheelchairs. We wanted to make sure that anyone in a wheelchair was properly included – there's no point in saying, 'Yes, you can come to prom in your wheelchair, but you won't be able to move from the table.') Anyone who had missed their own school prom could apply, but we also had requests from three 13 year olds with terminal illnesses who knew they wouldn't live to 16. That was a shock.

I'm always moved by the stories I hear through Friend Finder. No matter how tough you've had it yourself, there is always someone facing a harder battle. Take the epileptic boy who applied: his seizures are so bad and so frequent that he hadn't been allowed to go to his school prom, and when his mum wrote to us, she wasn't hopeful that we'd say yes either. I told her that we would find a way. And we did. We tracked down a folding screen so that every time he had a seizure, his mum could put the screen up to give them some privacy until it had passed.

If you think getting dressed up in fancy clothes and having a dance doesn't sound important, then that's because you've never had to sit at home on your own while your friends party, or lie strapped to a monitor in a hospital bed while your classmates head off for a night out. People assume that I arranged a prom because I'd missed my own, but that's not the case – when I first started planning the Friend Finder Prom I thought I was going to mine. I arranged a prom because they're fun – and being disabled should never be a barrier to that.

The work I was doing with Friend Finder and the prom was making me more and more aware that being disabled shouldn't be a barrier to anything, and that people like me could do anything our non-disabled peers could do. I decided that I would mark my sixteenth birthday by making a video saying exactly that.

My Top Tips for Life

* When you've got a goal, make a plan. I started planning the prom in total chaos and I was so disorganised that it could have very easily fallen apart. Start by making a list of what you need to do and a timeline of when you need to do it. Then put it on the wall. It will help you stay focused and not get distracted.

* Never be afraid to ask for help – it's not a sign of weakness, it's how you learn.

* At the end of each day, make a small note in your diary or notebook of what you have achieved that day, and also a list of what you need to do tomorrow.

* Always take time to acknowledge your successes and everything you've achieved so far, but don't let that moment of success distract you from the end goal – because that's where you're heading. A high point is just a service station where you refuel along the way.

GOING VIRAL

On 17th March 2017 I posted the following message on Facebook:

'Today is my sixteenth birthday. Please help me celebrate by watching and sharing my video to raise awareness. Thank you from Lewis.'

The video itself lasted for one minute 42 seconds. This is what I said:

'My name is Lewis Hine. I was born in 2001. At 17 months old, I was diagnosed with a brain tumour and it changed my life forever. I have had 13 brain surgeries to stay alive. I also have drug-resistant epilepsy and hydrocephalus and I have seizures most days. My life is a challenge. But one I am willing to accept. People say I'm disabled as if it is a bad thing, but I say I'm lucky. I know what my challenges are. I never take anything for granted, I don't feel sorry for myself, I use coping mechanisms to help me. In fact, I founded a project, Friend Finder, to help children who miss a lot of school come together to make friends. My project Friend Finder has now helped hundreds of children make friends. Disability isn't a bad thing, BUT keeping silent about it is! Today is my sixteenth birthday and I would like you to help me celebrate by sharing this video to show to the world that it's OK to be different. My illness may define the length of my life, but it won't define how I live it. My disability gave me the ability to understand and help others. And now I finally feel like I am living.'

I had no expectations when I pressed *share*, and I certainly didn't plan to make a viral video; I simply wanted to mark my birthday in a way that felt honest. But when I woke up the next morning, I discovered that it had been viewed over a million times. Messages were coming in from all over the world. There were tens of thousands of them and most were thanking me for bringing the problem of isolation to the world's attention.

There were messages like these from parents:

'Wow! My daughter is about to turn eight. She has

battled a brain tumour since she was eight months old. I am so pleased to see your positivity and light. I will tell her about you.'

'Happy birthday! My five-year-old son has intractable epilepsy too, Dravet syndrome. He misses a lot of school and your programme will be so great for him when he gets a little older. Thank you for sharing!'

'I cannot wait to show this to my son, who is 13 and faces his own challenges... I hope it will help to teach him to appreciate and be grateful for everything that we have. That ability (to be grateful and see the glass as half full!) is a huge, invaluable gift. Thank you for sharing it with all of us!'

'Love this. My son misses a lot of school due to having Noonan syndrome, always has. He has always struggled with making friends and developing those friendships for various reasons, ie bullying and attendance at school. "Friend Finder" is a fabulous idea. Happy Birthday Lewis!'

I had messages from other disabled young people too. Those really hit home. There was a girl in Pakistan, for example, with cerebral palsy. She wrote that before she saw my video, she'd pretty much come to the point where she wanted to end her life, because it was so difficult having an illness like that in her culture. The video, she said, had made her realise that she wasn't alone after all, and that gave her the strength and belief to go on. I found that really inspiring. She's stayed in touch through Friend Finder and I heard recently that she's started running quiz groups for other disabled kids in her area. She loves it, apparently, and it's helping her to say positive.

Discovering 50,000 messages in your inbox is a lot for a 16-year-old kid to deal with – especially one who struggles with his reading. I'm not going to lie, my first reaction was to stay in my room and hope it would all go away. But once I'd calmed down, I realised that these messages proved that I wasn't alone, and that there's a definite need for Friend Finder.

The message that has stayed with me most was from a little boy with a brain tumour. He was only four or five and he called his tumour his 'naughty bean'. He said, 'I've got a naughty bean in my head like you Lewis and I'm going to be big and strong like you. I'm not going to let my naughty bean get to me.' It really made me laugh, and the next time I went into hospital I thought about what he'd said; it cheered me up just like my video had cheered him up. And that's the thing, people think all the Friend Finder stuff is about me helping other people, but they help me just as much.

By 20th March the views had hit three million and I'd made the lead story on the *BBC Hampshire News*.

'Teenager's Facebook birthday video goes viral,' ran the headline, next to a huge picture of me. If that was a surprise, what happened next was unbelievable.

Mum and I were just sitting chatting in the kitchen when the Friend Finder phone rang. (We don't have an office but we do have a separate number for Friend Finder.) Mum picked it up.

'Hello, I'm trying to get hold of Lewis Hine,' a woman said. 'I work for Elton John. He's seen Lewis's video and wants to talk to him. How do I make that happen?'

Mum pulled her amazed face at me. 'Just tell Elton to ring my mobile,' she told her, and gave out her number.

We sat there for five minutes, waiting. I assumed it was some kind of joke, but Mum wasn't so sure.

But then her phone did ring. She gave it to me – and Elton John was at the other end.

'Hello, Lewis,' he said. 'I watched your video. I was so moved by it and it made me feel so good about everything in life. I just wanted to tell you that I think you're amazing. You're doing something so special for people. You have no idea how inspiring you are. To me, in this day and age when we have so much bad news, it's so wonderful to see someone so young doing something so brave and so wonderful. It teaches us all a lesson.'

I was so shocked to find myself on the phone to Elton

John at all, let alone have him paying me compliments, that all I could manage to say was, 'Just hearing that makes me feel so happy.'

'You make me happy by doing something so beautiful and so brave and so wonderfully moving,' he replied. 'It's just really inspirational to talk to you. I'll be in touch by email.'

And he was.

Well, after that, things just went crazy. Mum came into my room at about 6am the next morning and woke me up with the words, 'Lewis, we've got a living room full of people and big cameras. They want to speak to you.'

I just hid under the duvet.

'You made the video!' she reminded me, chuckling as I tried to get my head around it all.

'I don't know what to do,' I told Mum. 'I didn't think it through!'

She literally dragged me out of bed, gave me a Friend Finder T-shirt to wear and pushed me into the sitting room. There must have been eight or nine people in there from the BBC, plus some people from Radio Solent. It's not a very big room.

'We want to interview you on *BBC Breakfast*,' someone said.

I didn't know what to think. Appearing on live telly

sounded really scary, but on the other hand, it would mean millions more people would hear about Friend Finder.

We were miked up and told to sit on our sofa and wait for our cue. It was so early that Chloe and Jess were still in bed. The TV people kept saying, 'Stand by, stand by.' Mum and I had no idea what they were on about. Then at 7.08am one of them got a message. 'No, hold fire. Martin McGuinness has died – we've been pulled.'

Well, I was gutted. I'd spent the last hour psyching myself up to do a live TV interview and now it wasn't happening because some Irish politician had died. Radio Solent went ahead with an interview, which was great, but it wasn't *BBC Breakfast*.

I went back to bed and the next thing I knew, Mum was waking me up again. 'We're going to Manchester,' she said. 'The train's in an hour.'

'What?' I asked, really confused.

'The BBC called again,' she told me, stuffing some clothes into a bag. 'They want to interview you in the studio first thing tomorrow morning.'

Who knew that so many people watch *BBC Breakfast*? When I sat down on the famous studio sofa on 22nd March to talk about Friend Finder, we'd raised about £1,400 for the prom. By the time I was back in the lobby 15 minutes later, another £3,000 had come in and the video had reached 30 million views. It was unbelievable. I remember sitting in one of the funny green sofa booths they have there with Mum.

'Emails and messages are coming in from complete strangers offering to help you out,' she told me. 'All these people are sending you such lovely messages. Facebook is going absolutely crazy. So many donations have come through... Do you think we're actually going to get enough money to do the prom? I think this is going to be massive, Lew. How do you feel?'

I know I should have said, 'Excited' – after all, in the last six days I'd been on the telly, I'd had 50,000 messages of support and talked to Elton John – but I was finding it all a bit overwhelming, to be honest.

'Scared,' I said.

But when I walked into Prom HQ a couple of days later and told the team that we'd hit our £15,000 target, everyone was so thrilled, cheering and hugging each other, that I couldn't help but feel better. We had all worked so hard for so long, begging favours from the council and caterers and members of the local community... and now, all of a sudden, we had a proper budget. It was amazing. That was the moment when we all realised that this prom wasn't just a crazy dream; it really was going to happen. And it was going to be great.

My Top Tips for Life

★ So many people try to fit in and change themselves to be like others, but we should all just be ourselves. Admitting to yourself who you really are is hard. Making my birthday video and telling the world I am disabled was embarrassing, and the reaction was even more embarrassing, but I'm happy being me. My disability makes me who I am, and I'm proud of that. Whether you are big or small, have hair or are completely bald, be proud to be you. I bet if you haven't got any arms, you can use your legs far better than anyone else and probably leave people in awe of you, so be proud. Yes, our disabilities make our life a challenge – but you can rise to that challenge. My mum doesn't have a disability in the formal sense, but she definitely goes a bit crazy sometimes worrying about me, money, bills and being a single mum, so she uses her experience to help others and that gives her something to be proud about. My sister Chloe isn't classed as disabled either, but she dresses funny and that makes her happy, because it's her way of being herself.

★ We are all unique; we all have our own challenges. Don't hide from them – use them! Remember, our differences are what makes the world so interesting and colourful.

MY BIG PROM

WE SENT OUT 150 handmade invitations that week – one for every young person who had applied. The range of disabilities was huge. We had autistic kids, kids hooked up to catheters and breathing apparatus, and kids with terminal illnesses. We had a full medical team booked for the night, but each young person had to come with their own carer. As disabled kids ourselves, we were used to the problems people like us face at public events, and we tried our best to eliminate as many as possible. We had a team of chaperones who would come and sit and talk to the children while their carers went to the loo, for example, and I managed to track down a photo booth with enough space for a wheelchair and two carers. We may have had to compromise on lots of the plans, like the supercars and the film premiere lights, but there was no way we were going to let anyone's disability prevent them from being fully involved. I was determined that no one was going to feel excluded.

As the acceptances came flooding in, it really hit me that some of the kids who were coming were very sick indeed. I didn't want any of the team organising the prom to be upset by what they might see on the night, so I invited Neil from the Stress Management Society to come and teach us how to cope with any stressful incidents.

He gathered us all together and told us to breathe in and out very slowly. 'Breathe,' he kept saying. 'Breathe.' Then he gave us each two sweets.

'Just eat the first one normally,' he told us. 'But with the second one, I want you to close your eyes and suck it really slowly. Don't think about anything except what it tastes like.'

We all did what we were told (except Jess who just went, 'Whatever. Why would I get upset by a disabled kid when I live with one?'), but I didn't have a clue how it was going to help us deal with kids having seizures. Still, no one did freak out on the night, so perhaps it worked after all.

Neil didn't charge us for his time, which was incredibly generous because he's a busy man and his advice certainly gave us some fun with Mum as well. She was super-stressed on prom day, and every time any of the Friend Finder lot saw her, we'd say, 'Breathe, breathe. Suck the sweet!' It made her laugh.

The epileptic boy who had the very frequent seizures was there with the folding screen we'd managed to get hold of. His mum was concerned about how other guests would react but, of course, no one took any notice because every single person there had a problem of some sort, or cared for someone with a problem. It was quite funny, seeing this screen popping up and down all night.

There was a girl who was waiting for a heart transplant who hadn't danced for six years (she certainly made up for it on the night); a transgender boy whose school had refused to let him wear a suit to prom because they said he was a girl; and an 18 year old in a wheelchair who also had a condition that meant her skin was very sensitive. It had been difficult finding a dress that wouldn't irritate it, but in the end we got hold of this fabulous red one that was big enough to pin to the back of her wheelchair and drape over her. She had feet a bit like mine too, overlapping and out of shape, but we managed to get hold of some gold shoes that we strapped to the bottom of her wheelchair so that she could just rest her feet on them. She looked beautiful.

I don't remember a lot about the night itself. I do remember walking from the Premier Inn to the Guildhall in my suit and my brand-new gold Versace trainers (the entire family had saved up to buy them for me – they were two sizes too big so there'd be room for growth), and I remember standing in the lift afterwards with a bottle of Shloer and a carton of cheesy chips, but a lot of what happened in the middle is a blur. I know I danced a lot and that I spent a long time at the sweet table – there was a giant Ferris wheel of sweets which a woman called Kelly generously donated after reading about the prom on Facebook. And I know I made a speech.

Everyone says they hate speaking in public, but it's no exaggeration to say that I'd almost rather have brain surgery than make a speech. It's not just shyness; my memory is so bad that no matter how much I practise what I'm going to say, I know that as soon as I stand on the stage, I'll forget everything. And there's no point in anyone writing my speech down for me because I can't read very well. Especially when I'm nervous. And the worst thing? Thinking about what an idiot I'm going to look when I forget my speech makes me anxious – and anxiety triggers my seizures. The idea of having a seizure on stage makes me even more anxious. It's not good.

I'm asked to speak in public quite a lot these days and most of the time I say no, but sometimes I need to do it as a way of saying thank you. The prom was one of those occasions. People had been so generous, donating money and clothes and food and decorations and, most of all, hours and hours of their time. The prom was only a success because of their support. So the least I could do was stand up and say 'Thank you'.

But when I walked on stage in front of all those people, nothing came out of my mouth. I just stood there staring at everyone for about 30 seconds. That's a lot of silence when there are 300 people expecting you to say something. Eventually my brain re-engaged.

'All I want to say is thank you, everyone, for coming tonight and enjoying yourselves and showing your support,' I stammered.

Everyone clapped and cheered and I got off that stage as fast as I could.

A few things went wrong on the night, of course. We forgot to cut the giant 15kg chocolate cake for a start (I shared it with all the volunteers the next day and, since there was enough for 300 people, I took the rest around to our neighbours), and Jessica managed to convince the DJ that it was OK to play the uncut version of a hardcore rap song. One minute we were all dancing away, and the next Mum was running across the room like Usain Bolt, screaming at the DJ to turn it off. It was hilarious.

The next morning I woke up and I couldn't feel my legs at all; it was as if they'd been amputated. It was my own fault; I'd been determined not to use my wheelchair on the night because I wanted to dance and be the cool kid in his gold Versace trainers who had organised a massive prom – not Lewis Hine, the boy with legs so weak he has to use a wheelchair. I know it sounds silly, especially when there were so many kids in wheelchairs there, but I'd been planning this night for a long time and that's the way I'd always envisaged it. The next day was horrible, really painful, but I don't regret the decision.

I'm still moved by the stories I heard that night. One of the girls who came died soon after, and her mum called us to ask whether her daughter could be buried in the dress she'd worn for the prom. There's only one answer to a question like that.

We gave everyone who came a pen and a white card and asked them to write down how they felt about the evening. Reading the cards back is a humbling experience. We kept them all. These are some of my favourites:

'I'm so happy to watch my three sisters have such a lovely night.'

'Thank you so much for finding me some friends.'

'Thank you so much for doing this prom! I honestly thought I would never go to one. Thank you for making the impossible come true. It's good to feel like a princess.'

'Thank you for tonight. I was so relieved to find someone else who knows what I'm going through.'

'My son spent so many years in and out of hospital. Tonight has meant so much to him.'

'I made more friends tonight than I have done in my entire life.'

'I watched my daughter dance for the first time in six years. It made me cry.'

I think the best comment of all was from Izzy, a young woman whose brain tumour had eaten away the side of her face. She'd had reconstructive surgery not long before the prom and this was the first time in her life that she'd had the chance to dress up. She wrote, *'It's so nice to see that there are other people out there like me and I don't have to give up hope and that it's OK to be different.'*

That's why I put on the prom – to prove that being different is good. It's why I do everything I do.

Izzy's story

I was four when I was diagnosed with a rare brain tumour. I underwent numerous surgeries, chemotherapy and high-dose radiotherapy. I went back to school when I was six, but it soon became obvious that my brain had been damaged and mainstream school wasn't for me. I started going to a special needs school when I was eight.

It is the best place for me, but going to a special needs school can make you really lonely. When I first started there, the school only had 12 pupils, ranging in age from eight to 18. There are 40 of us now, but the age limit has increased to 20 so there are still very few students that I can call my friends.

I have lots of multi-disciplinary hospital appointments every year and I still have to be seen at the Royal Marsden every four months for an oncology check-up. I've had over 80 operations in all.

My older sister did a prom at 16 and 18 and it has been my ambition to go to one myself for such a long time. Mum found out about Lewis and Friend Finder on *BBC News* and then got me to like his page. When he posted the message about the prom, Mum sent an email straightaway.

Going to the prom changed my life completely. It was the first time I'd got to dress up and play princess and it made me realise that I'm not the only one who is lonely and feeling sorry for myself – there are others like me around, too.

Callum's story

I have something called fetal valproate syndrome (FVS). It has things in common with autism. I also have attention deficit hyperactivity disorder (ADHD), which means that I struggle to manage my emotions. I've recently been diagnosed with depression, too, which causes me to self-harm when I'm stressed.

I had really poor social skills when I was younger; I wanted everyone to be my friend and if I felt rejected for whatever reason, I would lash out. I threw things, swore and, in extreme cases, I'd have a total meltdown, banging my head on walls, rolling into the foetal position on the floor or under tables and crying uncontrollably. That could go on for as long as 25 minutes. I have had lots of support over the years and I'm happy to say that I can now control my emotions a lot better. I haven't had any extreme outbursts since I was at primary school.

I went to a mainstream school until Year

10, but I struggled to cope in large classroom situations so I moved to a specialist school to give me a better chance to succeed academically.

I missed loads of school because of my emotional and social difficulties and I really struggled to socialise. Before I came across Friend Finder, I spent most of my time at home. Then, in October 2015, my mum saw a post on Facebook advertising a Halloween party for children and young people who struggle to make friends because they miss a lot of school due to illness or disability, and thought it would be a great thing for me to go to. I had a really good time. It was great to be able to have fun with other kids like me.

Friend Finder has been brilliant for me. It's helped me with my social skills, and the parties and outings mean that I now have somewhere I can go and be myself, where I don't have to worry about what other people think of me. It has also given me a better understanding of the challenges other kids face in life.

Saffron's story

When I was 13, I developed an autoimmune disorder called post-streptococcal disorder, which means that when I get a cold caused by streptococcal bacteria, the antibodies that are produced start to attack my body – in particular my brain, heart and eye muscles. It has also caused reactive arthritis, which means I have difficulty walking. My immune system is also weak, so I usually spend most of the winter months ill and off school. Some of my summer holidays were spent in hospital having and recovering from surgery.

This illness has also left me with chronic fatigue syndrome which means that I find doing normal things like going to school extremely tiring. From the age of 13, I could only manage to be there for half the day. I also had to reduce the number of GCSEs I took. Never being in school at lunchtime meant that I missed out on chatting to my classmates; I found within a term that the friends I'd made at school had forgotten I existed.

I wasn't able to go out because I couldn't walk very far, which made it hard to see my friends from outside school who were all starting to be more independent. A friend did introduce me to a girl called Katie who lives nearby, but as we both have chronic illnesses we rarely got to meet up!

Life is lonely when you're sick, and most people can't understand the difficulties we have just trying to do ordinary things that they take for granted. I hate making plans too far in advance as I know that the chances of me being well enough to follow through aren't great. And even if I am, I get tired very quickly. I also have to be really careful in the winter because there's such a high risk of me catching another infection that will take months to recover from. I spend a lot of my time on my own.

I first heard about Friend Finder through Katie. Her sister had been in contact with Lewis and she asked if I would be able to go to the prom. It was amazing to be invited. I didn't think I would be well enough to go to my school's prom on my own and I didn't really want to be the only girl with her mum tagging along!

I found out about Friend Finder once I had been invited to the prom. My condition is a rare one (affecting around one in 100,000 people), so there aren't any support groups and it is very isolating when there is no one that really gets it. Meeting Lewis and lots of other children who can relate to the same things as me was so lovely and it has made my world a less lonely place. Including all children regardless of their 'condition' is something that was missing, and it's given me a lovely group of friends who 'get it'. I'm really looking forward to helping Lewis and the rest of the group with the next proms!

My Top Tips for Life

* We all have our own challenges in life. Every single one of us has our own story of things we've been through. The trick is to use those experiences and feelings as fuel to help push you forward. I chose to use my fuel not only to help me keep fighting, but to help others keep fighting, too. Friend Finder and the prom gave everyone the opportunity to make friends and experience a night to remember forever. I used my disability to understand and help others just like me. I changed my story by following my dreams and working hard – and you can too, whether you're like me, struggling to be seen, or a parent or sibling feeling helpless as you watch your family member suffer. We may not be able to change our prognosis or the length of our life, but we can certainly change how we live.

* You can volunteer, help others, or challenge policies and old practices that no longer reflect today's needs. Doing things like that will not

only give you a positive focus but when you achieve your goal, you'll feel like you've made a difference. You can't restart your story, but the next chapter is still to come and it's up to you what happens next.

★ I use this thing called 'positive affirmation' to help me achieve my goals. When my sisters and I were small, my mum gave us all a small cardboard box. She told us to paint them and put something that represented our dreams inside. Back then, I put a toy car inside mine, but as I got older, she explained what the box really meant and how I should use it. My dream became my goal. I put in a piece of paper with these words written on it: 'Helping others makes me feel great.' I would look at my piece of paper every night and say the words out loud.

There was also a second piece of paper that said, 'Standing in my drive next to my Lamborghini and looking at the massive house I've just bought makes me feel proud.' But that's one of the chapters that hasn't happened yet!

I know it sounds crazy but trust me, it works. Reading your goal every night means that you don't forget it in the business of daily life. Stay focused on your goal, work hard and you're halfway there. Try it for yourself. Get an affirmation box (or get one for your child or family member) and read your goal every night. Imagine that you've just that second achieved it. Think about how it feels. Hold on to that feeling and let it inspire you to carry on. Let me know how you get on!

★ I know exactly how I'm going to feel when I get my Lamborghini and big house. I visualise that moment in my head and I look pretty good if I'm honest (lol).

A Day in the Life:
23rd January 2018

7am: Early start today. I hate waking up early but I have to go to Great Ormond Street and we're catching the train. I take my meds.

8:30am: The train's packed full of business people and there are people standing right down the carriage. Lucky we booked a seat.

10:30am: We're here. We took a taxi from the station because the tube was really crowded.

11am: I'm in the scanning department as I have to have an MRI today. They're putting a cannula into my arm so they can put some dye into my body to help with the pictures they're taking. They've just asked Mum if she could be pregnant, as the dye is radioactive. That really made her laugh.

An MRI scanner is really scary. It's a long tunnel that you lie in for ages and it's so noisy that you have to wear big headphones to protect your ears. They strap your body to keep it still and because they're scanning my brain, I have to have a cage over my head too. There is a small mirror in the cage so I can see my mum, who's sitting by my feet wearing matching headphones. Once I'm ready they move me into the tunnel. I used to panic and have to be put to sleep, but I've had so many MRIs now that I'm OK with it.

12:30pm: I was in the scanner for over an hour today. I'm exhausted – if you move at all they have to start again so I have to concentrate really hard.

4:30pm: We're finished at the hospital so we start our journey home. I'm tired and the train is packed again and this time we don't have a seat. We move to the disabled reserved seats but they're full too. We are standing in the aisle and there's a pregnant woman standing with us as well. My disability is hidden so people wouldn't necessarily know I need a seat, but even if they did, I doubt anyone on this train would move. They're not getting up for a pregnant woman, after all. Mum and I decide to sit on the floor.

7pm: Home! Jess and Chloe tell me what

they've been doing all day. They definitely
had more fun than me, although Jess did get
stuck on the school bus for an hour after it
broke down on the way home. She couldn't
call Mum to pick her up as she was in hospital
with me, so Jess just had to sit and wait for the
replacement bus. I tell her at least she had a
seat. She doesn't think it's very funny.

9pm: Mum's given me my meds and thinks
I'm in bed but I'm on the Xbox, lol!

11pm: I'm watching a film in bed. I think
today's stress has taken it out of me because
I'm not feeling too well and I sort of know
tonight's going to be rough. I feel funny, like
I often do before seizures, but there's nothing
I can do to stop them. I'm a bit scared to be
honest.

9

EVERYONE NEEDS
BACKUP

THREE WEEKS after all the excitement and glamour
of the prom, I was back in Great Ormond Street
Hospital. It was a planned visit, one of the two or three
monitoring sessions I have each year when they take
me off my meds and study my seizures.

I think the planned hospital visits are worse than
emergency admissions – at least when I'm rushed in,
I know my life's being saved and I leave feeling better.
Invasive monitoring or, in this case, video telemetry,
are just exploratory and I come home exhausted.
So walking up to the hospital entrance on that June
afternoon felt a bit like approaching the gates of hell. I

may have been wearing my Versace trainers, but it was a far cry from the red carpet at the Guildhall.

Video telemetry is when your brainwaves are videoed over several days using a camera. After I'm shown to my room – which is just big enough for a single hospital bed, a chair and a tray – I get into bed and a doctor comes in and glues electrodes all over my head. (Once they're on, my whole head gets covered in a big white bandage which ties up under my chin, so it looks as if I'm wearing a bonnet. Cool or what?) The wires from the electrodes are then plugged into the wall and that's me stuck. I can't move from my bed until the tests are over. They go on for a week. Oh, and a nurse has to put a cannula in my arm, too – that's a tube stuck into a vein – in case I have a seizure I don't come out of on my own and need an intravenous injection of rescue meds. There's always a risk of that happening (Mum has a bottle of the muscle relaxant Midazolam at home for emergencies), but the chances are much higher when I'm off my epilepsy drugs.

And then the tests begin. Anyone who's had video telemetry will tell you they're torture. Like the invasive monitoring, this whole process is about trying to find the bit of my brain that's responsible for my epilepsy, so the doctors need to see what goes on inside my head while I'm having a seizure. The trouble is, seizures don't happen to order, so the doctors do all these things to bring them on. Like put huge lights right up close to my face and shine massive strobes in my eyes, or get me to breathe in and out really fast like I'm hyperventilating. My seizures are also triggered by having to think about more than one thing at a time, so they ask me maths questions and make me play board games too. I had a massive seizure playing Monopoly once, so that now seems to be their favourite; just seeing the box makes me want to snap the board in half.

So, it's fair to say that Great Ormond Street was about the last place on earth I wanted to be at that moment. Though ironically, I'd pretty much asked to be there. Earlier in the year, I'd gone in for an assessment and my consultant had basically told me that the tests were a waste of time. She didn't put it quite like that, of course, but she did say, 'There's nothing more we can do, Lewis. You can either accept that your seizures aren't going to get any better and stop coming for these tests, or you can carry on. It's up to you, but if you keep coming you must understand that we can't promise that anything will improve.'

I didn't stop to think. I just said, 'I want to keep trying.'

I meant it – giving up isn't on the cards for me these days – but as I felt each electrode being stuck to my head, I wondered whether I really had made the right decision.

And to make matters worse, it was the night of my school prom. I know I'd just organised one of my own, but it was still hard to see the messages and photographs coming in on social media as my classmates got ready. I decided to ask my Facebook friends to cheer me up.

'So, I'm back in hospital,' I wrote. 'I'm here all week having tests and I already feel tired. I'm connected to a monitor which means I can't leave my hospital bed, or at most a few feet around it. I'm not looking forward to this and I know that I'm just one of thousands of children today feeling like this. This is exactly the reason why I launched Friend Finder, so kids like me don't have to feel isolated while we're in hospital. I know as the week goes on that I'll get worse, so I need to stay positive. I have an idea. Can you go to a window, or anywhere if you're outside, and take a photo of whatever view you can see and share it? I may be stuck in a room with four walls, but maybe you can be my eyes. Share this post and help me see the world from my hospital bed in London. Tag other poorly children and adults as well so they can see the views around the world too.'

The response was amazing. My post was eventually viewed 38,000 times. I was sent pictures of a back garden in Surrey, a grizzly bear in Alaska, a lemon tree in Peru, a field mouse in Australia and a group of postmen and postwomen outside their depot in New Milton, Hampshire, each holding a piece of green paper with a letter on it. The message read, 'Best wishes Lewis Hine.' It must have taken ages to organise. I couldn't believe they'd gone to all that effort for me.

Seeing all these pictures made such a difference to how I felt. They gave me the push I needed to keep positive.

And so did Mum. Again. It's not an exaggeration to say that I couldn't do anything without her constant support. I might not be a little kid anymore, but Mum never leaves me when I'm in hospital. She sleeps on a pull-out camp bed in a curtained-off area at the side of my room when I have to stay in overnight, and she sits on the end of the bed when I'm in the MRI scanner. These days I'm so used to being in the tunnel that more often than not I fall asleep, but it's good to know she's there.

I come from a big family – as well as the four of us, there's Nan and Grandad, four uncles, one aunt and ten cousins. We all live within five miles of each other and Mum and I know that we could call any of them at any time. Mum had to ask my Uncle Ritchie to help us get from Great Ormond Street to Waterloo station once. She couldn't manage me, the wheelchair and the suitcase all on her own, so Uncle Ritchie came up to London to help her. There's a family Facebook page that Mum uses a lot when she's worrying about me in the middle of the night.

My nan and grandad are incredibly supportive. Discovering that I had a brain tumour hit them really hard. Nan practically lived in the hospital chapel – she lit so many candles the priest came in and told her, 'He might survive the operation, but he won't survive the massive fire you'll start with all those candles.' Grandad said he'd sell the house if he had to. He would have done, too.

Then there are my sisters. I described them as irritating when I was asked about them in the video Radio 1 made for the Teen Award, and they are. They tease me all the time, calling me the 'favourite child', and Jess has been known to raid my chocolate supply; but they are also a massive part of my story.

They never let me feel sorry for myself, for a start. Chloe will come into my room if I'm feeling a bit down, and literally drag me out of bed. 'Come on, Lew,' she says. 'Come on!' She won't take no for answer, so there's no point in arguing with her. It's a tough approach, but it works. Chloe's been a bit of a role model for me, to be honest. The way she dealt with being bullied at school is one of the reasons I'm doing what I'm doing now.

And they have been forced to become young carers because of me. If Mum has to go out, one of them has to stay in. Chloe's 18 so she does the most. She took me to the dentist recently. It was the first time she'd taken me out by herself and I know she found it hard. She had to do everything for me, from opening the car window (it's an old car so has a handle rather than a button) to helping me walk into the surgery. And when I got there, I couldn't remember whether I'd used the special mouthwash, so she had to phone Mum. She was exhausted by the time we got back.

Jess is only 15, but even she has to help me sometimes. I wanted to buy Mum a surprise Christmas present last year and Chloe was at work. It wasn't just because I might get lost or have a seizure, I also needed Jess to look after the money and help me at the till. It was nice that she did it – usually Mum has to buy her own present from me and pretend to be surprised – but, let's face it, it's a bit weird having to ask your younger sister for help with something as simple as shopping. It does bother me that she's more capable than I am.

Having a disabled brother has a huge impact on their lives. They've had to put up with endless cancelled outings and holidays because I've been ill, and suffer more embarrassing incidents than anyone should have to go through. Like the time I managed to wee all over the car (I was only five), or when I had a major seizure on the London Underground. We were all standing, and when the seizure started, I threw my head back so violently that I head-butted Mum. Then I collapsed on the floor and everyone was staring, wondering what was wrong with me. When the train came into the station, people just stepped over me. Mum, Chloe and Jess had to make a wall around me. I wet myself then, too, apparently.

And of course, I take up most of Mum's time. She wouldn't admit it, but I think that's really affected Jess and made her do things to get some attention. She had a massive house party when I was in Great Ormond Street a couple of years ago. When Mum and I got home the next day, there were doors missing, the loft hatch had been torn off and the hall floor was completely ruined. Somebody had covered it with washing-up liquid, got the hose from the garden and turned it into a slide. It was like a scene out of that film *Project X*.

When Mum opened the front door, she just stood there with her mouth open.

'It wasn't me,' Chloe said, running down the stairs.

Then Jess appeared from the living room. 'Well, you wouldn't want me to throw a lame party, would you?' she laughed.

That did it. Mum stared at her. She was so furious she could barely speak. 'Too soon,' she whispered. 'Just get out of my sight.'

I wasn't all that bothered about the doors and the floor, but I was really worried about my room. Luckily for me no one had touched it – it was the only room that hadn't been trashed. I think they were scared of all the medical equipment in there – it was the first time in my life I felt glad to have a bedroom that looks like a hospital.

Jess is an absolute legend around here now, but Mum won't leave her in the house with just Chloe any more. When Mum's away with me, Jess has to go and stay at Nan and Grandad's.

I'm pleased to say that they do all get some time off. Chloe's at college studying music technology, Jess goes to school and Mum receives ten hours a week respite care, courtesy of social services. She gets to catch up on sleep and I get to be looked after by Matt. He's 25 and a rapper in his spare time. Mum was really keen to find me a young male carer because I spend so much time with her and my sisters. She doesn't think that's good for me.

Matt's a laugh, more like a friend than a paid carer. One time he took me to a fair and he and his friend Joe started chucking all this face paint about. I ended up with a great big blue stripe across my face and Matt was covered in glitter. It was really funny. Another time he took me out for a burger in a pub and when we got home, he said to Mum in this serious voice, 'I'm afraid we had to leave early because Lewis got into a fight.'

Mum totally fell for it. 'What!'

We just burst out laughing.

Doing stuff like that makes me feel normal.

So you can see that I depend on a lot of people. I need them to help me physically and I need their emotional support, too. Knowing that Mum, Chloe, Jess, Nan, Grandad, Matt and the rest of the family are on my side and are willing me on is the main reason I'm able to achieve my goals. They were all there at the prom, for example. I could hear them cheering while I stood like a lemon on the stage trying to remember what I wanted to say. I'm lucky to have them.

I like to think that it's not totally one-sided though. Now that I've started to be invited to cool things like backstage meetings with famous rappers, Mum, Chloe, Jess and I have made it a rule that we do everything together. We're a team.

My Top Tips for Life

* I talk a lot about how important family is, but family doesn't just mean your blood relations. A family is the people who are there for you when you need them, who help you because they care about you and not because they want something in return. Not everyone has a mum or dad and there are lots of children with no brothers or sisters, but there are two kinds of family: the one we're born into, and the one made up of people we find as we go along. We call them friends, but if they stick by you, they're family. A good friend will be in your life forever.

* Never judge a book by its cover. My mum says that to us constantly. It means take the time to get to know someone before deciding you won't get on, because first impressions aren't always right. You don't have to be friends with everyone – we're all different, right? – but sometimes people can surprise you. And when you do find a friend, make sure you're there for them.

10

RECOGNITION

'WE WON!' I posted on Facebook on 22nd June 2017. It was late and I was in bed, but Friend Finder had just been given its first ever prize – the Digital Leaders 100 Mobile Innovation of the Year Award – and I couldn't wait to share the news. It was a big deal – we'd been up against nine others, including the global mobile advertising and discovery platform InMobi and NHS 24's Step It Up Scotland.

When I walked on stage to collect the award, the announcer said that Friend Finder had won because of the way we had taken existing technology, in the form of Pokens, and used it to help change the lives of people in the local community. Hearing that made me really proud – not that the other 499 people in the room would have realised that! Instead of making an emotional speech naming all the people who had made it possible, all I did was mutter, 'Thanks.' It was a black tie dinner and I wasn't even wearing a tie when I accepted the award.

I admit that it was hardly my finest moment, but I wasn't feeling well. We'd had a stressful day. I'd woken up with a bad head and aching muscles and by the time Mum, my wheelchair and I made it to the St. Pancras Renaissance London Hotel (which looks like something out of Harry Potter, by the way), I needed a sleep. But I'd barely closed my eyes when Mum discovered that she'd forgotten to pack my smart trousers. It was 4.30pm. The champagne reception started at 6.30.

'Quick, Lew,' she said. 'There are shops in St Pancras station. We'll have to go buy some new ones.'

There was only one pair of black trousers to be found and they were miles too long. I was ready to give up, but Mum persuaded the shop assistant to tape the hems up for us. We didn't have time to wait while she did the actual taping, so as soon as she'd pinned them to the right length, Mum and I went back to the hotel to get changed. Or half-changed – I had to keep my shorts and trainers on, which looked a bit weird with a dinner jacket and tie. Then Mum ran back to the shop, pushing me in my wheelchair, and I put the trousers on, crossing my fingers that the tape would hold, Mum stuffed my shorts and trainers into her handbag and we arrived at the reception just in time. Mum looked like she'd been dragged through a hedge and my head was banging.

When we looked at the programme, the Mobile Innovation Award was one of the last.

'You're not going to make it to the end of the night, are you, Lewis?' observed Mum.

I shook my head.

She went off to speak to the organisers and they agreed to change the running order so that the Mobile Innovation Award could go first. The woman Mum spoke to told us later that it had caused a bit of a panic – apparently they'd wanted Friend Finder to be the big finale. Trust me to muck things up!

It was hot in that room and, since I didn't think Friend Finder had a hope in hell of winning, I started to take off my tie as the shortlist was read out. Big mistake. I'd just got the knot undone when the announcer said, '... and the award goes to Friend Finder!' Still, at least my taped-up trouser hems didn't fall down.

It's not every day that my condition affects a grand three-course awards dinner in a posh London hotel, of course, but it does have an impact on my own and other people's lives on a daily basis; and, as Friend Finder has become better known, that impact has become increasingly public.

Two days after the Digital Leaders 100 Awards, I was due to give a TEDxTeen talk at indigo at The O_2, a venue next to the O_2 arena. It holds over 2,000 people and the talks are also streamed live to 150 countries around the world. I hate public speaking, as you know, but I said yes to this because TEDxTeen is the perfect audience for Friend Finder. The TEDxTeen programme was set up to enable communities and individuals who are interested in social action to have conversations and connect. The theme for that day was 'Bold Moves' and I'd been asked to speak about the bold move I'd made when I posted my video and told the world that I was disabled.

There was a rehearsal the day before, but I had a massive seizure in the car on the way there and by the time we arrived, I was in no fit state to do anything but lie down. The organisers had given us a family room at the Intercontinental so we went straight there, which pleased Mum and Chloe because they love staying in hotels. When the guy came to ask if we needed anything, Mum was so excited she said, 'It depends. What do you have that's free?'

He thought that was really funny. 'Quite a lot,

actually,' he laughed, to which Mum replied, 'Well, we'll have one of everything that's free then, please.'

I was really embarrassed, but he came back ten minutes later with this tray piled up with stuff – toothbrushes, razors, slippers – which I must admit was pretty cool.

I wasn't feeling much better when I woke up the next morning, and I could barely speak when we got to the indigo. It was obvious that I wouldn't be able to give my talk. Mum went to speak to the organisers and they agreed that, rather than not do anything at all, they would play the birthday video. When my turn came (there were other speakers, including a Syrian refugee who became a UNICEF ambassador of education and a young woman who set up an anti-bullying app), someone stood up and said, 'Today's theme is Bold Moves and today Lewis has made the bold move of admitting that he is too ill to do his talk. Sometimes the biggest challenge is admitting that you can't do something.'

I was really touched by that, and when the video ended I got a standing ovation. I hadn't had to say anything. Result! It's not often that being ill actually works in my favour.

Not long after that I had a seizure at an awards ceremony. I'd been made an #iwill ambassador (#iwill is a UK-wide campaign that aims to make social action part of life for as many 10 to 20 year olds as possible by the year 2020, and is co-ordinated by the charity Step Up To Serve), and on Wednesday 22nd November 2017, I was one of 50 ambassadors lucky enough to be invited to this big celebration at the Tower of London.

I was having a rough week. A couple of days earlier I'd had a seizure so violent that I'd fallen into the telly and smashed it (I don't often break things, luckily), and then I had two more on the way to the Tower, so it was hardly a surprise when I collapsed again.

We'd just been shown into this room where we were supposed to relax before the ceremony started. Mum has two criteria for calling an ambulance when I have a seizure: blue lips, or a seizure that goes on for longer than five minutes. This one ticked both those boxes, so she dialled 999. I remember the paramedics were really excited.

'We've never been to the Tower of London before,' one of them said, as he strapped me into the wheelchair (the room was two floors up so they had to carry me down to the ambulance), 'it makes a change.'

That made me laugh – I may have caused a scene and missed out on getting my certificate, but at least I'd given the paramedics a day to remember.

They sent me the certificate in the post. Because I have both the memory of a goldfish and a proud mother, it's stuck up on my bedroom wall, next to the Points of Light one that arrived out of the blue on 17th July 2017. That day, I'd been sitting on my bed playing on my Xbox when Chloe came in holding a white A4 envelope. It had '10 Downing Street' printed across the top.

'What is it, Lew?' she asked, once I'd got it open.

I scanned the contents, bewildered. 'Seems to be a letter from the prime minister,' I said. 'Can you tell me what it says?'

'Sure!' said Chloe excitedly, and began to read it out: '"Dear Lewis, I want to congratulate you on becoming the UK's 724th Point of Light. The Points of Light Award recognises outstanding volunteers who are making a real difference in their communities. You are changing lives through Friend Finder and the Friend Finder Prom, helping to provide a supportive network for young people with illness or disability. Your work has inspired millions and has done much to raise awareness of the loneliness faced by young people battling long-term illness. Up and down the UK volunteers like you are helping to build a country that works for everyone. The Points of Light Award is a small thank you on behalf of the whole country in recognition of your exceptional service. Best wishes, Theresa May."'

I just sat there, while Chloe shouted for Mum and Jess. 'Hey, come in here. Guess what, the prime minister's written to Lewis!'

They rushed in, half expecting it to be a wind up. I showed them the letter.

'Wow, that's brilliant Lew,' they laughed and gave me a massive hug.

'I really don't know what to say,' I stammered when they finally released me. 'I'm shocked – the prime minister has heard of Friend Finder! That's really made my day.'

I haven't put my GCSE certificate up on the wall. I've always known that I'm never going to be a rocket scientist and my results prove it. I got a U for religious education, an E for food tech and a grade 1 in both English and maths. Most people would have been devastated, but I hadn't been expected to get a grade at all in English, so you could say there was something to celebrate.

I was disappointed with my food tech result, though. It was my favourite subject at school and I was pretty good at the actual cooking bit. Obviously, I can't follow recipes and I need other people to chop things for me because I'm not really safe around knives, but with a bit of help, I can create tasty dishes. I had to make lasagne, noodles, pizza and chocolate mousse for the GCSE and my family scoffed the lot as soon as I got it home. I pretended to mind, but it felt like a real achievement.

My grades weren't anywhere near good enough to get me into sixth form college but luckily for me, the head thought that all the things I was doing outside school were as impressive as lots of exam passes, so he let me in. The first couple of weeks were tough – there are 4,000 students there and I had no idea what to expect – but once I'd settled in, I really began to enjoy myself. It was so different from secondary school – no one seemed bothered by the fact that I use a wheelchair sometimes, and if anyone mentioned my scar it was just to ask what it was from; once I'd explained, that was it. Some people had seen the birthday video and had heard about the prom, but it wasn't a big deal. I was just another ordinary student and that was exactly what I wanted.

Things did change a bit after the TV documentary *My Big Prom* went out on 14th November 2017 as part of CBBC's *My Life* series. There was a lot of media attention afterwards and the college posted a link to the documentary on their website, so it was hard to stay anonymous. But although I was dreading going into college afterwards – I'd been seen on national TV in my pyjamas, after all – everyone was really supportive. Lots of people came up to talk to me about it, and most of them offered to help with the next two proms.

I didn't get to watch the documentary live because I was doing a radio interview about it for BBC Radio Solent at the time, but we did a big screening of it later that evening and invited all the volunteers who had helped to come, too. It was a weird experience to see everything we'd done over those months documented on the telly. Watching it made us all realise what a massive team effort it had been, and how much we'd accomplished together. A lot of people cried that night.

The day the documentary screened was especially crazy. That morning I'd been in London being interviewed on *This Morning* with Phil and Holly. They had asked Izzy, one of the guests from the prom (you can read her story in 'My Big Prom'), to come too, and we'd all stayed the night before in London. We had to get up at the crack of dawn and when we got down to the hotel lobby, we found that ITV had sent Izzy and I separate cars to take us to the studio. We felt like proper celebrities! We were taken to make-up as soon we got there. I hate having to wear make-up; they have to put powder on your face to stop you looking all shiny, but it feels gross. Then we were shown into the Green Room. That's a waiting room, basically, and we walked in to find a bunch of fashion models, ten puppies and Kelly Brook in there already. I managed to grab a selfie with Kelly.

I don't mind doing live telly. I know it sounds crazy for someone who says he hates public speaking, especially when you think how many people are watching (around a million people tune in to *This Morning* every day apparently); but it's the idea of an audience in front of me that freaks me out, and the great thing about telly is that you can't see anyone except the people interviewing you. Izzy was really relaxed, but Mum was so nervous she didn't say anything unless she was asked a direct question.

The response to the CBBC documentary was amazing. I'd done interviews about it on *BBC Breakfast*, Radio Five Live and *Newsround* the day before too, as well as an interview for the digital and online radio station Fun Kids that I had to do in a cupboard at the *This Morning* studio. (I was so busy that the interviewer from Fun Kids agreed to talk to me while I was waiting to go and talk to Phil and Holly. The cupboard next door to the Green Room was the only quiet place we could find!) By the following week the Friend Finder GoFundMe page had received £3,000 in donations.

I know I've said it before, but people's generosity is incredible. That money will be used to help fund the next proms, which are being held in Portsmouth and Birmingham. Two is a lot to take on, but so many people contacted me after the first one, asking if there was something similar happening near them, and saying that I had to expand. And we are a bit more organised this time – there are two planning committees and several team leaders who'll be in charge of different areas, like dresses or fundraising.

Friend Finder has become an official registered charity since the prom, too. It took ages because, quite rightly, the Charities Commission want to know everything from your safeguarding policies to how you do your accounts. But on 2nd November 2017, Mum had an email from them. It read, 'We are satisfied that Friend Finder Official is a charity and it has been entered onto the Register of Charities with the Registered Charity Number 1175539.' I was so proud that I printed it out and stuck it on my bedroom wall with the other certificates.

The decision to apply for charity status was a tough one, because once you become an official charity, you no longer have complete control. Before, I could decide to hold a Friend Finder swimming day or a fundraiser at Portsmouth's Spinnaker Tower, say, and I could just go ahead and do it (the fundraiser raised £5,000, thanks to brilliant auction lots like 'Spend a day as CEO of Portsmouth Football Club' and Mum's auctioneering skills). Now I have to run every idea by the board of trustees first. That does slow things down, but the massive upside is that it means I've created a legacy. Now that we have serious professional people to help us – like Donna Jones, leader of Portsmouth City Council, the brilliant businessman Paul Barham, IT specialist Jock McEwan and event management superstar Zoe May – I know that Friend Finder will always continue, regardless of how well or ill I am. They all say that as the founder, I'm still top dog, but it doesn't worry me either way. What matters is that we now have expert help. And seeing as I told an audience of about a million on *This Morning* that I plan to take Friend Finder global and I have no idea how to do 99 per cent of the stuff that this entails, I could really use some help.

My Top Tips for Life

My life is constantly throwing up new and unexpected challenges. I'm terrified half the time, but I refuse to give in to the fear since it's part of making Friend Finder a success. This is how I prepare before I have to do something I'm scared about:

★ I talk it through with someone, usually my mum. I tell her how I'm feeling and she helps me get it all into perspective.

★ I draw a picture that represents how I feel. (I draw because I have trouble writing, but you could write it down or just make a mark on a piece of paper. As long as you know what it means, that's all that matters.) Then, next to it, I draw a picture of something that makes me happy, like my Xbox or my dogs, Poppy and George. I find it helps to connect something I like with something I'm worried about. Sounds a bit crazy, I know, but it works for me.

★ I don't want to let my fears control what I
do or don't do, so I've decided to take each
request as it comes and give it my best shot.
After all, the things we worry about are
usually less scary in real life than they are in
our heads, so the best way to get over them is
to face them head-on.

NEXT STOP, THE WORLD

'WAKE UP, LEW!' Mum said – too loudly – as she turned on the light. I groaned. It was still pitch dark outside. 'Come on. We've got a plane to catch.'

Then I remembered. We were going to Hawaii. Mum didn't need to tell me again: I was already up. The trip wasn't a holiday; I was going – along with Mum and Jess (Chloe couldn't get time off college) – because in September 2017, I'd been made a Bakken Invitation Award Honoree. The award was set up by the medical device manufacturer Medtronic to recognise people who've overcome health challenges with the help of medical technology, and who are using their 'extra life' to help others. The programme is named after

Medtronic co-founder Earl Bakken, who says that medical technology – a pacemaker, insulin pump and heart stents – have given him ten or more years of extra life to give back to society and make a difference. Mum had read about it somewhere and decided to nominate me. It's a worldwide programme and the panel only select 12 honourees each year, so it was a bit of a long shot; but since the prize was a $20,000 donation to a charity of your choice (that's around £14,500), plus an all-expenses-paid trip to Hawaii to participate in community service projects and workshops, she thought it was worth a go. And the gamble paid off. We were chosen.

Which is why Jess and I found ourselves squashed up against her suitcase in a taxi at 6am on a freezing morning in January 2018. I was excited about the trip, but travelling is always a hassle for me. There's all the luggage, for a start. As well as normal stuff like clothes, we have to take my wheelchair, a rucksack full of meds (we have to carry those with us because we can't risk them getting lost somewhere en route) and another cabin bag with spare clothes for me in case I have a seizure. Try navigating your way through a busy airport with that lot.

Sitting still for long stretches of time makes my back hurt, so we'd decided to break the journey in LA. That's over 11 hours on a plane, and by the time we arrived I was exhausted. And a bit confused; LA is eight hours behind the UK time-wise, so it was still only 3.30 in the afternoon. I felt like I'd been in a time warp.

Some things stay the same however far you travel. Like people shoving in front of you to get on the hotel shuttle bus, as they did at LA International Airport. We were near the start of the queue when the bus drove up, but we still ended up missing it because no one had the patience to wait for the driver to lower the wheelchair ramp. We'd have missed the next one, too, if an off-duty pilot hadn't turned up and held the other passengers back. Then, when we finally made it to the hotel, we saw that the entrance was three steps up from the pavement. There was a lift up to the entrance (basically a metal box, minus a lid), but none of the hotel staff seemed to know how to open it. Then, when someone did eventually get me inside, it got stuck and I was left sitting there like a lemon while they tried to fix it.

That kind of stuff happens when you travel in a wheelchair, and I try not to let it get to me. Travelling is hard but life is for living – that's my motto. I may have been trapped in a lift, but at least the lift was in LA!

The next day Mum hired a car and drove the three of

us to Hollywood, which was pretty cool. It's not every day I get to pose for a photo on the Walk of Fame, or shake hands with a life-size Oscar statue. I felt like the luckiest person alive.

But what happened two days later pushed my – and Mum's – patience to the limit.

We were back at the airport for the onward flight to Hawaii. Mum had booked assistance and a lovely woman took us over to security, where we joined the queue for the X-ray machines. Jess went first but when it came to me, we were told that no one was available to search me in my wheelchair; so the assistance person just parked me to one side and told me and Mum to wait.

We did. For ages. Mum was stressing about Jess, who was on her own on the other side of security. Eventually one of the airport staff came up to me and said, 'Can you get out and walk?'

'I suppose so,' I shrugged.

Mum wasn't happy about it. 'He had a seizure not long ago. He's not very strong.'

The guy just looked at us. We didn't want to risk missing the plane, so Mum helped me up and I followed her through the scanner. My legs were so weak that once we were through, I had to hold on to Mum and Jess while we waited for my wheelchair. Loads of people were watching and I got a bit upset, especially when Mum had to help me put my shoes back on. It was embarrassing being stared at. My mum's pretty cool, though, and she just told me to take a deep breath and move on.

By now I really needed to pee. We looked everywhere but there didn't seem to be any disabled toilets. Mum asked several airport staff, but they all told us the same thing: 'The disabled cubicles are located inside the ladies' and men's toilets.'

'Well, which one do we use then?' Mum asked. 'I have to help him.'

A security guard did offer to take me into the men's himself, but that was no good because I need Mum's help to actually use the toilet.

'In that case, there's a separate disabled toilet in the next terminal,' said the guard. 'It's about a 20-minute walk from here.'

I couldn't hold on for another 20 minutes. I was bursting.

Mum could see that I was getting upset.

'Jess, stay with Lewis,' she said, marching off into the ladies. She came back a couple of minutes later. 'I've asked every woman in there whether they'd mind if I take you in and they all said no,' she told us. 'So come on.'

There were about ten women in there when Mum pushed me in. Everyone smiled, but no one really took much notice of us, which was nice. But as Mum pushed my wheelchair into the cubicle, she burst into tears. 'Why does everything have to be so hard?' she cried.

I didn't know what to say. I felt really sorry for her.

When we came out, Jess told us that she'd overheard a group of airport staff talking about what Mum had done, saying she shouldn't have let Lewis use the ladies and that she'd caused a scene.

Hearing that brought Mum back to her usual tough self. 'Forget it,' she said, blowing her nose. 'Let's all just take a deep breath and move forward.'

We went off for a big American breakfast of waffles, bacon, cheese, Boston baked beans and pancakes. It was delicious and cheered us all up, but inside I was really angry. I posted a long message on Facebook when we got to Hawaii, describing exactly what had happened and tagging both the airport and American Airlines before I pressed send. This is how the post ended:

'This morning is one of the few times my disability has really affected me and my family and it was just because of other people and their lack of knowledge of what it's like to be disabled. I won't let this ruin my trip, I will have a great time but I say to these companies, please be educated in the fact that not all disabled people have same-sex carers, and separate disabled toilets give all the amazing disabled people around the world like me some dignity.

'I would like to invite the executives of both American Airlines and Los Angeles International Airport, and any of their staff too, to come and join me for a day in a wheelchair to help them understand how they can ensure all their customers have a good experience from the moment they arrive at the airport to the moment they fly out.

'Please share this post to raise awareness of this and hopefully get it changed. Our disabilities make life colourful, they give you the opportunity to think outside the box and be creative and make a difference to help everyone. Please take this opportunity so I don't have to nearly pee my pants in public again. From Lewis ☺.'

The post was shared 400 times. Most of the messages that came in were from those who'd experienced the same kind of discrimination, but quite a lot were from people saying they'd never thought about the difficulties disabled people face in their day-to-day lives before, and now they would. I never heard anything from the airport or the airline, but I did get a message from an architect who designs public buildings promising to take what I said on board. That felt good. Change happens one small step at a time.

Just 24 hours later, we were watching wild sea turtles in a lagoon in Hawaii. Mum and Jess were in the water, pushing me in a kayak, and the sea turtles were swimming around no more than a metre away from us. They kept bobbing their heads out of the water, like they were saying hello. We tried to be as quiet as possible so we wouldn't disturb them, but inside we were all bursting with excitement. You never get to experience anything like that in England. I could hardly believe I was there.

I could have spent the whole week watching them, but we were here to work. As Bakken Invitation Award honourees, we were expected to take our social action projects forward, and the purpose of this week was to teach us how to do that. There were talks and workshops every day. In that first session we had to imagine that we'd all been given a canoe. We were then told to picture our end goal and describe how we could use the canoe to reach that goal. When my turn came, I said, 'My goal is to take Friend Finder global. I don't have time for a canoe. I need a rocket pack!'

Everyone laughed (and I was known as 'rocket boy' for the rest of the week), but I meant it. I want Friend Finder to reach every corner of the world and I want it to happen fast.

And it turned out that this trip to Hawaii has

provided the fuel for that rocket pack because it gave me the chance to connect with so many brilliant people. The other honourees came from all over the world. There was Claire from Ireland who set up the Scoliosis Advocacy Network; Clarissa from Uruguay who's helping to educate people about diabetes; Jason from New York, founder of type 1 diabetes organisation Marjorie's Fund; Lindsay, another New Yorker, working to raise awareness about sudden cardiac arrest; Hui, who's working with the Bethune Charitable Foundation to expand access to healthcare services back home in China; and Ismael from Mexico, who volunteers with two Parkinson's support groups. He was there with his friend and care-giver Diego, and they made us laugh so much. One day we met them in the breakfast room and when we asked them where they'd been the day before, they said, 'On a helicopter tour. We're in Hawaii!' We got on really well with Clarissa and her husband Alejandro too – he had helped Mum get me in the kayak so I could go and watch the sea turtles.

These are just a few of the amazing people we met, and they'd all won the award for creating inspirational social action projects. Everyone was so warm and supportive of what I'm trying to do with Friend Finder that I went back to England feeling I was so close to reaching my goal I could almost touch it. Both Clarissa and Claire said that a lot of the children they work with would really benefit from Friend Finder and have encouraged me to expand the charity in Ireland and Uruguay; Hui promised to do everything he could to help bring Friend Finder to China; and I'm already talking to Diego and his 19-year-old daughter Adriana about holding a Friend Finder prom in Mexico. I am determined to use the connections I've made through the Bakken Invitation to take Friend Finder global so I can help people like me all over the world.

I also left Hawaii knowing that I was one step closer to achieving another goal. That $20,000 grant will pay for almost an entire prom, and another AV1 robot like the one I'd received in the summer of 2017. AV1 is the first telepresence robot (that is, one that helps people to take part in events remotely) to be made specifically for kids with long-term illnesses and disabilities. It works with wifi or the 4G network, and is controlled via an app on your phone or tablet. Once your AV1 is turned on, you can move its head using the touch-screen app, see through its eyes and communicate with whoever's nearby via the microphone and loudspeaker. It was developed by No Isolation, a Norwegian company who create tailored communication tools that help tackle loneliness, and it's designed specifically to help its users stay connected with school and their friends.

When No Isolation sent us the first one, I started using it to help me at college. It now lives in the classroom during the week; when the teacher does the register and discovers I'm not there, she gets it out and sits it on my desk (it's less than 30cm high). If I'm feeling up to working that day, I turn it on via my iPad and then I can see and hear everything that's going on. (Its eyes and head light up so the teacher can see I'm joining in with the lesson.) If I want to ask a question, I just press a button on my iPad and the AV1's head blinks white lights. It's just like me putting my hand up. If I'm not feeling so well, I press another button and the head turns blue to show I'm listening, but not up for answering questions. And when my friends go for lunch, they take the AV1 with them. It's made a massive difference to me: I miss fewer lessons so I'm learning more, and I can be part of college life even when I'm at home or in hospital.

AV1 is just perfect for Friend Finder and so my other goal is to get 100 of them for Friend Finder to use. It's a big ask because this kind of technology doesn't come cheap. Even with my terrible maths, I know I need to raise serious money. But you don't get anywhere if you don't think big.

I took my AV1 with us to Hawaii and we did a presentation with it – we got Jess to sit out in the corridor with the iPad while Mum and I stood in front of everyone with the robot.

'Jessica isn't here,' Mum explained, 'but thanks to AV1 she can see you and hear you. So – wave, everyone, and say hello!'

I think Jess must have been really embarrassed, because when everyone had stopped waving and shouting, there was a long pause and then this really tiny voice just whispered, 'Hello.'

We were lucky Jess didn't say anything controversial.

The day before we'd used the AV1 to play this really hilarious trick on Mum. We were meant to be rehearsing for the following day, so she'd gone downstairs to the presentation room with it, leaving Jess and me in the bedroom with the iPad. The app was on and we could see on the iPad, through the robot's camera, that Mum was walking along the corridor towards the lift. A man walked past her: it was just too good an opportunity to miss.

'Hello, sir,' we said into the iPad.

'Hello, sir,' went the robot.

'Shush,' Mum hissed into her bag where she had put the robot.

The man gave her a funny look, and then Jess added, 'Hello, hottie!'

That made him really stop and stare. Thanks to the

robot's camera we could see that Mum had gone bright red. 'Oh my God, sorry! It's the robot,' she told him. 'In my bag.'

He just hurried away – you could see he thought she was completely crazy. Jess and I were in hysterics as Mum tried desperately to zip her bag closed to shut us up.

I had a perfect opportunity to show off the robot the next morning. There was a networking breakfast with all the top guys from Medtronic, including the chairman and CEO Omar Ishrak, and I was planning to talk to him about sponsoring an AV1. My idea was that companies could pay to have their logos printed on its chest. But before I had the chance (I'd just sat down with my French bun – imagine an iced bun, only heated up), everyone's phone pinged with the same message:

'Emergency alert.
Ballistic missile threat inbound to Hawaii.
Seek immediate shelter. This is not a drill.'

Then the hotel's siren went off, and the TV news on a screen at the back of the room was interrupted with an emergency notice:

'A missile may impact on land or sea within minutes. This is not a drill. If you are indoors, stay indoors. If you are outdoors seek immediate shelter in a building. Remain indoors well away from windows. If you are driving, pull safely to the side of the road and seek shelter in a building while lying on the floor. We will announce when the threat has ended. This is not a drill! Take immediate action measures.'

It was like the world had suddenly gone mad. Somebody shouted at us to stay where we were, because we were next to the ballroom – also the hotel's bomb shelter, apparently. But Mum took no notice of everyone else. She grabbed my arm and started dragging me towards the door.

'Jess is upstairs,' she was saying. 'If we're going to get blown up then I want to be with her.'

I was so shocked, I just followed her without a word.

There were people running in all directions but Mum was just ploughing through them all. She'd stopped being a normal mum and had turned into a power machine.

Finally we got to Jess, who'd seen the text message but hadn't really registered what was going on until we burst through the door shouting, 'Jess, where are you? There's a missile! We're going to get blown up!'

Then Mum pulled us both close to her and took us back down to the ballroom. As we were all huddling together around a table, I realised that this so-called bomb shelter was actually an open-air ballroom; it didn't have a roof. That's when I started to believe we really might be about to die. I know it sounds strange – you'd think we'd have been running around screaming, but now Mum had got Jess and I together, we just sat there waiting for the missile to hit. I think we were too shocked and terrified to talk. I certainly was. I clung on to Mum, who was desperately attempting to get hold of Chloe in the UK, but she couldn't get a signal. That really upset her – she was dialling the number, repeating, 'Chloe, I have to speak to Chloe.' Lots of other people in the room were doing the same, trying to get hold of their families. Jess looked as cool as cucumber on the outside, but I could tell that even she was panicking inside – she kept looking round at everyone else to see how they were dealing with it.

Exactly 38 minutes after the first text, everyone's phone pinged again.

'NO missile threat to Hawaii.'

It was over. We were safe. Most people in the room cheered and hugged each other. I had a massive seizure and vomited all over the floor. Mum had to stay and sort me out, but Jess went straight back upstairs to tell her friends at home all about the latest drama.

We found out later that an employee at Hawaii's Emergency Management Agency had pushed the wrong button when he was coming off shift. Some mistake!

Still, it got us on *BBC Breakfast* again. Someone had spotted my post about the (non) missile attack on Facebook, and that evening the three of us did a live interview with presenter Ben Thompson from our hotel bathroom. (The light was better in there.)

When Ben asked Mum about what had happened, she came across as calm, but actually she'd been shaky and upset all day – I think all the effort of getting me and Jess in one place and worrying about not being with Chloe had really got to her.

Then Ben turned to me.

'Maybe you could explain a little about why you're there?' he asked.

'I'm in Hawaii to receive an award,' I replied.

'For?'

'Charity work and stuff like that,' I said, tongue-tied. It was a massive opportunity to plug Friend Finder, but I'm afraid I blew it. All I could add was, 'Obviously no one expected things to turn out how they did.'

I was still a bit freaked out, to be honest. I'd spent

most of the morning asleep, recovering from the seizure, so I wasn't thinking straight. Never mind. Loads of people saw the interview and we had all these messages saying, 'Only you could go all the way to Hawaii and end up on the telly!' That made us laugh.

Later that evening, I got to meet Earl Bakken, the man who founded the award. It was incredibly inspiring to talk to him. He's in his nineties and in a wheelchair and is the most amazing philanthropist. He knew all about Friend Finder. That made me so proud.

As he shook my hand and gave me my Bakken Invitation Award medal, I promised myself that I would use this honour to make *him* proud, too, of what his award had made possible. I also found myself thinking back to something Mum had said in the presentation we'd given the day before (she spoke because my nerves had got the better of me again): 'Friend Finder is something that started from a small idea in a bedroom. Now it's actually changing people's lives.'

It's true. There's so much more that I want to do, but standing next to Earl at the end of that totally surreal day, I realised that I have laid a path, with the help of everyone who has supported and believed in Friend Finder. And now all I need to do is walk it. How exciting is that?

My Top Tips for Life

★ Travelling can be hard for anyone, but if you have an illness or disability, it can throw a whole new set of challenges at you. So don't be afraid to ask for help or advice. Always call the airline or travel company in advance to see how they can support you.

★ Make sure you have enough medication for the trip, plus a few extra days' worth in case you're delayed. If you're travelling to somewhere in a different time zone, ask your doctor when you should take your medication, especially if you're epileptic like me.

★ Plan some rest days when you don't do too much, so you can really enjoy the days you do go out. Everyone feels better for a break.

★ If you come across things that make your life more difficult than it should be – like I did with the toilets in LA airport – let me know via Friend Finder (Friendfinderofficial.com).

Companies won't know there's a problem unless we tell them, so let's tell them. Every change starts with a single idea or one voice; don't be afraid to be that voice.

★ When you're travelling, don't spend the entire time with your head in your phone or iPad. Look around you – the world is amazing.

★ If you ever find yourself in the middle of a missile crisis, make sure the bomb shelter you're hiding in has a roof! And when your life flashes before your eyes like mine did, make sure the show's worth watching.

★ Wherever you are, remember to look at the stars!

A Day in the Life: 5th February 2018

9:30am: Mum has just woken me up. I get the feeling she's been trying to wake me for ages because she was almost shouting, 'Come on, Lewis!' I tell her I'm too tired to get up and that my back and legs really hurt, but she reminds me that I have to go to Great Ormond Street Hospital today for a brain scan.

10.34am: We're on the train from Havant to London Waterloo. It's a pain being in a wheelchair because you have to ask the guard to get a ramp and let you on, and then you have to hope that no one's sitting in the space reserved for a wheelchair. It's quite a big space so people often put bikes and things in there.

12 noon: We've arrived at Waterloo. We're both hungry, so we head to Marks and Spencer for a sandwich and packet of crisps. We've given up trying to use the tube – it's just too hard in my wheelchair, and even when I'm walking it's too hectic for me – so we go and find a black cab. Mum asks the driver if

he minds if we eat our sandwiches in the back
and he says it's OK. We start chatting and I
tell him about Friend Finder. He sounds really
interested and when we get to Great Ormond
Street, he says, 'Black cabbies often help with
things like this so if any children from London
are going to the prom, I'm sure I could get
some drivers to take them for free.' Then he
rips off the corner of a newsletter and gives it
to me. It's the contact details of the black cab
central office. How nice is that!

12.40pm: It's strange heading into Great
Ormond Street. It's totally familiar, of course,
but I don't come here for fun so it also brings
back lots of memories of pain and nasty tests.

2pm: I'm getting ready to go into the MRI
scanner. Today's scan is a bit different: it's
called a 'language brain scan' and there's
hardly anywhere you can have one done,
apparently. The doctor told me that people
come from all over Europe to have one. It's to
try and help my epilepsy because my seizures
are getting worse. I have to meet with a
neuropsychologist first; she explains about the

language games they're going to do with me while I'm in the scanner, so they can see how the part of the brain that controls my speaking and listening reacts. She tells me the sorts of questions they'll ask, but I don't understand a lot of them. She says, 'Answer the question with a verb,' but I don't know what a verb is. Then she says, 'What do you think of when I say cat?' I can't think of anything, which makes me feel really stupid. Mum's helping to explain – she says, 'Say meow or stroke,' but I just don't get it. There are too many questions and the neuropsychologist is asking them too fast. I don't like it.

4.30pm: I'm feeling pretty fed up. I was in the scanner for ages today and my back was hurting so much that I found it even harder to concentrate than usual. Mum's doing her best to cheer me up but I really don't feel like smiling.

5.30pm: We finally leave the hospital and Mum takes me straight to Starbucks for a treat. I have a hazelnut latte and a toastie.

7pm: We're back at Waterloo and ready to

go home. The train journey is only about 1 hour 20 minutes, but I'm really tired. I feel a bit guilty because I can just close my eyes and go to sleep in my wheelchair while poor Mum has to stand, but I don't have any energy. The train is so packed that people are standing in the aisles and holding onto anything they can. It's crazy.

9pm: Home! Mum's helping me get ready for bed. I'm not sure why, but my body keeps shaking. I just tried to eat some noodles but my hand was wobbling so much that they kept falling off my fork, so Mum had to help. It's horrible. I feel dizzy, too. Mum thinks it's stress and since my head doesn't hurt, she's not going to take me to hospital. (If we went every time I was ill, we'd live there.) She gives me my meds and helps me into bed. I'm feeling pretty pants. I have to go back to Great Ormond Street in two weeks' time for a whole week of tests. I know hospital is a necessary part of my life, but that doesn't mean I have to like it. I don't normally let hospital and my illness get me down but I'm tired tonight and not feeling too good. But I'm sure things will be better tomorrow.

OVER TO MUM

BEING A MUM is the best feeling in the world. Carrying a child for nine months, helping them to grow in a safe place inside you where you are able to protect them and keep them warm until they are ready to be born into the big wide world is an incredible experience. Once they take their first breath, they are vulnerable to everything, and from the day they are born they start their own journey – their own life.

I've had three children, and Lewis's birth was the easiest. He was a dream child, smiling and laughing all the time. But at 17 months his life took a change of direction: when he was diagnosed with a brain tumour, it was devastating. I had spent the previous year and a half stopping him from bumping his head or scraping his knee and now, with no warning or time to adjust, I was having to hand my child over to a complete stranger, knowing he was going to remove part of his skull and cut into his brain.

The guilt you feel when your child is sick is overwhelming. I kept asking myself what I'd done wrong. Why was Lewis so poorly? Was it my fault? At that moment it took all my strength just to stand on my own two feet. How, I wondered, is any human being supposed to cope with a situation like this and not curl up in a ball and want to die?

I soon discovered how. You cope because you have to. Yes, you're suffering the most horrific pain inside, but you have to be the strongest person on the outside to keep everyone else going. Lewis needed me to be strong for him, so I put my own fear and tears away and threw myself into being the best mum I could be, for him and my girls. I promised myself that I would give them the best life I could and that I would always support and be there for them, no matter what.

When Lewis came out of hospital two weeks later I was a nervous wreck. He looked like Frankenstein's monster with a head covered in stitches and I held him as if he was made of glass, terrified I would break him. This was the start of 16 years of living under a constant cloud of fear and on a rollercoaster of uncertainty. I would wake each morning wondering whether today would be the day he didn't come round from his seizure, or would crack his head open during a fall. Or perhaps it would be just another day of watching him struggle with normal life, smiling from ear to ear and completely determined to live the amazing life he wished he had. The fact that his life was so crap but he was always so happy regularly broke my heart, and there were days when I would lock myself in the bathroom and cry. I felt so guilty that my son had such a hard life. He was in constant pain and could only dream of doing what his sisters or other children did. Being a mum is amazing, but being the mum of a very poorly child is far more life-changing than normal parenting. With a healthy child, things get easier as they get older and start to look after themselves, but when your child has an illness, they don't; things are hard every minute of every day.

When Lewis told me that he wanted to start fundraising for charity I almost couldn't believe it. My first thought was, how can someone who goes without so much want to do things for others? But he did. The atmosphere at his first ever fundraiser, where he bowled against the world champion, was electric. Every person there was just having fun and feeling good in the knowledge that they were helping others. Lewis was only three years old, but he still gave a press interview to the local newspaper and television. He just thanked everyone for coming and said he was raising money for the poorly children and ASBAH, but it was amazing. He was the smallest person in the room that day, but he was by far the most powerful – a small youthful voice that captured everyone's attention. I realised then that whatever Lewis lacked in physical ability, he certainly made up for in mental ability and understanding of others. It was obvious that he could make his voice heard and that there was something very special about him that made people want to help him.

He used that ability as he grew up. A bowling fundraiser turned into an army of superheroes running the Great South Run and many more events. He had raised over £20,000 for charity by the time he hit his teenage years. Supporting Lewis and his ideas hasn't always been easy. Fundraising for a cause, organising events and now running his charity Friend Finder for him has been an incredible learning experience for the whole family.

As you'll have read, Lewis's story is not as simple as 'Lewis was sick, then got better, did some fundraising and became a hero'. The truth is that his condition isn't curable, and he spends a lot of his life either in his hospital bed at home feeling unwell, or actually in hospital. His shunt keeps him alive but if it blocks, or gets infected, then he's in a life-or-death situation. As he was growing up, I had to learn how to spot the difference between a childhood illness and a blocked shunt. I knew that getting it wrong could make the difference between Lewis being alive or Lewis being dead. That's quite a responsibility for someone with no medical experience. It was very stressful, but I soon discovered that a mother's instinct is a real thing and that I could trust it. In fact, on a few occasions, that instinct saved Lewis's life.

One day in 2009 the school called to say that Lewis had a headache and could I come and pick him up. This was nothing unusual, I had calls like that most days, but when I got there, Lewis was asleep on a bean bag in his quiet room. I put him in his wheelchair and took him home. Lewis said his head really hurt, so I lay him on the sofa and got him some painkillers and a glass of water. I wrapped his favourite blue Power Ranger blanket around him and waited to see if the painkillers worked, but after 20 minutes the pain was worse. He said that he felt sick and couldn't see properly. I knew it was his shunt. I called the hospital and they told me to bring him in straightaway.

When we got to hospital they gave Lewis a CT scan,

and a registrar we'd never met before told me that the results showed the ventricles in his brain were OK, so they didn't think his shunt was blocked. (Ventricles carry the water in the brain and usually swell when his shunt blocks.)

There was a swine flu epidemic at the time and every patient admitted into hospital was automatically tested for it. A blocked shunt has many of the same symptoms as swine flu and so, when Lewis's scan came back clear, that's what they assumed he had. He was immediately put into the side room on the neurological ward and kept in isolation. A few hours later, I was told that he was being transferred to a special swine flu ward and that's when things started to go a bit crazy. I could see that his scan looked OK, but somehow I just knew that it wasn't flu, it was his shunt. I also knew that if they moved him to the swine flu ward they'd be putting him in danger. He would probably catch it and, with his existing medical problems, that could kill him. I wasn't prepared to take that chance so when they came to move him, I barricaded the two of us into the room and refused to let anyone in. One of the top hospital executives was called to the ward. He explained, through the shut door, that they had a new protocol in response to the outbreak and that it was very important that they moved Lewis to the containment ward. I suggested he come in to talk rather than shouting through the glass, but he refused. He was worried about getting infected. I knew Lewis didn't have swine flu, so I told the executive that if he wanted to talk to me, he had to come in. Several minutes passed and then there was a knock on the door. I opened it to find both him and a ward nurse standing there, gowned up from head to toe with matching aprons and face masks. They looked pretty scary. I sat opposite them in my unprotected jeans and jumper and explained that until the test came back as positive for flu, I wanted them to listen to my concerns and stay open to the idea that Lewis's shunt might be blocked. I didn't want to cause trouble, but I could see Lewis was in terrible pain; I knew that if his shunt was blocked, his brain was being crushed, and while bureaucracy and drama were taking the focus away from his condition, he could be dying in front of me.

But they wouldn't listen. They left the room and started to make arrangements to move him. So, when the nurses changed shift, I kidnapped my own son. I took him out of the hospital in his wheelchair and left a letter on the bed explaining why I'd done it. The letter also made it clear that I wasn't going to bring Lewis back until the swine flu results were in and I could be sure that he would get the right treatment. What the hospital staff didn't know was that we were just sitting outside in the car. I was so worried about Lewis that I didn't want to leave the hospital grounds.

The ward nurses called me, but I told them that I wouldn't bring him back until I knew they were going to make him better, not worse. Then they called my mum and my brother Mike to see if either of them knew where I was, and suddenly my phone was ringing non-stop with people looking for me. I was so scared. I had taken Lewis out of the hospital without telling anyone, he had cannulas in his hands and feet, he was in terrible pain but no one would help me and no one would listen. I knew I sounded like a mad person, but I also knew that it was his shunt that was the problem and I couldn't give up.

Eventually the consultant called me and said that they had the results: Lewis did not have swine flu. Within minutes I was back on the ward and they put a bolt in Lewis's head to measure the pressure in his brain. It was sky-high. Lewis was rushed into surgery to replace his shunt and save his life. As soon as he was safely in the operating theatre, I collapsed on the floor and cried. The fight and exhaustion had scared me forever.

Lewis's life is a constant balance between life at home and in hospital; when he was 14, he really started to struggle with the feelings of isolation caused by all the time he'd spent away from school. When he came up with the idea for Friend Finder I was in awe of him. He put so much time and energy into the planning. His daily seizures and headaches would make most people feel sorry for themselves, but Lewis fought against all that and was constantly pushing forward to help more and more disabled children like him, so that they too could make friends and not experience the feelings of loneliness that he'd grown so used to.

There is so much that Lewis can't do, but he still founded a national charity because he wasn't afraid to ask for help. A lot of people find asking for help a sign of weakness or defeat, but in fact it's a sign of strength. Lewis began to learn so much, and because he knows he has the memory of a goldfish, he asked me to document and take photographs of everything he was doing to help him remember.

When Lewis won the Radio 1 Teen Hero of the Year Award, I was so proud I thought my heart was going to burst. My daughters and I were in the audience watching. One of us had to walk to the stage with him, and I just assumed that it would be me. But as it got close to the time, I was so worried that I'd burst into tears of happiness and pride that I had to ask my eldest child Chloe if she'd take him instead. I didn't want to upset Lewis seconds before he walked onto the stage at Wembley. Chloe agreed, but when his name was announced and I looked out from the audience, I could only see Lewis walking bravely and proudly on his own onto the stage in front of 10,000 people. When we all met up afterwards, Lewis said, 'Well, that was embarrassing! By the time we got to the stage door Chloe was crying so much she couldn't walk, so I left her there in a heap of tears being comforted by the stars from *Made in Chelsea,* and walked onto the stage by myself. I told Nick Grimshaw about it as we came off together, and he laughed, but what was even funnier was that when we walked around the corner, Chloe was still there in the same spot, and she was still crying! Nick gave Chloe a big hug and we all went off laughing. Next time I'm taking Jess!'

I guess that shows how proud we all are of Lewis. We see him fight every day to do the most basic things, like getting up in the morning and getting dressed; so to see what he has achieved over the past years makes us very emotional. The fact that he's helped so many people at such a young age is amazing, but if they could see the reality of his daily life they'd realise that he is a true superhero. That's why I was so proud when he was asked to write this book; it's a chance for him to finally tell his inspiring story.

I have learned so much from Lewis's humility and

kindness towards people. His passion and drive inspire me when I'm feeling down. His fighting mentality and determination never to give up keep me going every single day. His disability gave him the ability to understand and help others, and it gave me the challenge of raising a family that sticks together through good times and bad: a family that faces adversity as a unit of strong human beings, helping others and living each day as if it were our last. Lewis may need a mechanical pump in his brain to keep him alive, require my constant supervision and have a massive impact on everything I can or can't do, but when you've grown a real-life superhero in your tummy, you can't help but watch in amazement and enjoy it with a massive smile on your face. I am so proud to be Lewis's mum! Lewis was born to be different, not because of his illness or disability, but because of his big heart and passionate vision to make the world a better place.

AFTERWORD

I STILL CAN'T BELIEVE that I was asked to write a book. To be honest, revealing the details of your private life to the world is pretty scary, and embarrassing at times. There were occasions when Mum got upset when I was asking her questions about what happened when I was a baby, which was tough for me to see; looking through all the photos choosing what to use was difficult too – I couldn't believe they were actually of me. But I'm hoping that by sharing my story I'll help others, and if my book makes a difference to just one person then I'll be happy. Making a difference to someone's life is all I've ever wanted to do.

I'm more determined than ever to keep fighting

and to achieve my goals. I want to make Friend Finder a global charity and make sure that every child suffering with an illness or disability anywhere in the world has at least one friend. I'm organising two more Friend Finder proms, but I want to do even more. There are children missing out on their school prom every year because they're too unwell to get there, which means that I need to help them attend one and feel special every year. I want to take the proms global, too; hopefully, the prom in Mexico that I'm planning will be the first of many around the world.

I want to give 100 children across the UK a robot so that they can continue to access education from hospital or their beds at home, and still feel included. I'm going to approach the government to ask if they will recognise that a child is in school if the robot they're operating is in their classroom. That recognition would have a really positive impact on the lives of children who, like me, are unable to go to school every day, and it will help schools too.

I want to work hard and achieve my goals so that hopefully, the Medtronic Foundation will invite me back to Hawaii, and I'll be able to share how I used the award as an incredible platform to take my charity global. I know that, with hard work and determination, anything is possible.

Writing this book has made me realise that this is just the beginning. I don't know how long I have on this earth, but I can promise you one thing: I'm going to make every day count. I want to travel the world and watch the Knicks play in New York, see a show at Caesars Palace in Vegas, try out surfing in Hawaii and go to the Paralympics to cheer on my peers. I want to learn how big charities become global and I want to beat KSI at FIFA. I want to have new experiences and help change the way people view disability everywhere. My illness gave me the ability to understand and help others, so that's exactly what I'm going to do. Life may have dealt me a challenging hand, but I'm not ready to fold yet. I'm proud of my disability and, for the first time in my life, I finally feel like I'm living.

ACKNOWLEDGEMENTS

I WOULD LIKE TO SAY a special thank you to my mum, Emma Hine, and my sisters Chloe and Jessica. Their lives changed forever the day I was diagnosed with a brain tumour, but instead of feeling sorry for me or themselves, they helped me to fight, and encouraged me to follow my dreams. They sat for hours and hours during the process of writing this book, helping me to remember things. I couldn't have done it without them.

Special thanks also go to the Sophie Hicks Agency and Bonnier Publishing for believing in me and giving me this opportunity to share my story with the world. I was a big gamble, as I can't read or write very well;

but with the help of the amazing Charlotte Abrahams, I've done it. Charlotte sat on the end of a Skype call or phone and listened to my voice memos for so many hours I lost count; she was brilliant at rearranging our meetings at short notice around my seizures, and always noticing when I was tired and needed to stop. It must have been challenging working with me and around my illness, but she did, and it's meant that my book has become a reality.

In addition, I would like to thank the following people for their valued contribution to my book: Nan and Grandad Bicheno, Uncle Richard, Mike, Stephen, Alan and Auntie Marie, Callum Austin, Saffron Barnes and Izzy Colville, Elton John, Kid Ink, Tha Alumni Clothing, Nick Grimshaw, KSI, Jennie Jacques, BBC Breakfast, Radio 1 and O_2.

I would also like to thank the following who have helped me on my journey. Without them, I wouldn't be here to write my book:

Great Ormond Street Hospital
 Dr Varadkar
 Emma Ninnis

Queen Alexandra Hospital Portsmouth

⋆ Acknowledgements ⋆

Southampton General Hospital, especially children's neurosurgery

    Mr Sparrow

    Dr Whitney

    Chrissy Ward

    Mandy, Kate, Shona and the amazing team at children's neuro

My healthcare workers, especially Matt Stevens

Roslyn Ferguson

Solent Mobility Centre

Tech21

Mark Smith and The Car Finance Company

ActionCOACH

Giant Leap Photography

Manic Stage Productions

Hotel Chocolat

The Digital Awards

Young Epilepsy

Philip Haynes

Leon Legge

Marks and Spencer

No Isolation and the AV1

CBBC

CTVC, especially Leonie, Will, Georgia and Emily

Portsmouth City Council

Portsmouth Guildhall

Poken

Medtronic Foundation
   Audrey, Jacob and team

O_2 and Mark Evans for believing in me, the amazing GoThinkBig team – Bill, Tracey, Kerry, Craig, Alex and Lilly – and the gang at the Think Big Hub

Ajit Sharma, Elliott Lenton, Chris Buggie and Adrian Cunliffe from O_2 Wifi for helping me meet Kid Ink

Gary Lockwood and 24/7 Fitness for supporting Friend Finder and always being there for me.

And finally, thanks to everyone who has attended a Friend Finder event. We couldn't have done it without you!

ABOUT THE AUTHOR

LEWIS HINE is the founder of the charity A World With Friends. He lives in Portsmouth, Hampshire with his mum and two sisters. This is his first book.

www.lewishine.co.uk
www.aworldwithfriends.com